Ch. F. Brunner B. G. Weber

Special Techniques in Internal Fixation

Translated by T. C. Telger

With 91 Figures

Springer-Verlag
Berlin Heidelberg New York 1982

Dr. med. CH.F. BRUNNER,
Professor Dr. med. B.G. WEBER,

Kantonsspital, Orthopädische Chirurgie, CH-9007 St. Gallen

ISBN 3-540-11056-9 Springer-Verlag Berlin Heidelberg New York
ISBN 0-387-11056-9 Springer-Verlag New York Heidelberg Berlin

Library of Congress Cataloging in Publication Data. Brunner, Christian Ferdinand, 1937– . Special techniques in internal fixation. Bibliography: p. . Includes index. 1. Internal fixation in fractures. I. Weber, B.G. (Bernhard Georg), 1927– . II. Title. [DNLM: 1. Fracture fixation, Internal – Methods.
WE 185 B897s] RD103.I5B7813 617'.3 81-16601 AACR2

Printed in Germany.

Reproduction of figures: Gustav Dreher GmbH, Stuttgart
Typesetting, printing, and bookbinding by Universitätsdruckerei H. Stürtz AG, Würzburg
2124/3130-543210

Dedicated to
Professor Dr. med. Maurice E. Müller

"And above all, there is no culture without freedom."
EUGÈNE IONESCO, 1979

Introduction

The development of internal fixation techniques as taught by the Swiss Association for the Study of Internal Fixation (ASIF)* in 103 courses since 1960, and as laid down in the *Manual of Internal Fixation* (MÜLLER et al., 1977), has had a worldwide influence on the management of bone fractures. Crucial to the success of these techniques are: (a) an appropriate indication, (b) observance of correct biomechanical principles, and (c) strict aseptic technique. If these requirements are met, good results are consistently achieved.

The ASIF technique evolved largely from the work of M.E. MÜLLER, former chief surgeon at the Clinic for Orthopedic Surgery of St Gall County Hospital in Switzerland. Its principles have been applied not just to fracture therapy, but also to reconstructive procedures in orthopedic patients. Since 1960, interfragmental compression, internal splinting, and their combinations have become standard surgical procedures, contributing to the solution of routine problems as well as more complex surgical challenges. The present book is concerned with internal fixation techniques to be applied in cases where the basic techniques are unsuitable, or, more frequently, where a more elegant solution is possible.

Every internal fixation should achieve maximum effect with a minimum of material and effort. In all the techniques described, the basic biomechanical principles remain the same. The reader may be surprised to learn that almost all the implants used have been derived from the standard instrumentarium. It is unnecessary to manufacture a special plate for every conceivable fracture situation; the ASIF principles, the basic implants and the corresponding operative skills are sufficient for almost any situation that may arise.

Unquestionably, certain of the techniques presented here are already practiced elsewhere. Guest physicians, participants in advanced ASIF courses, and publications may have contributed to this. In writing this book, our object was not to lay claim to originality, but rather to demonstrate the freedom for creativity, modification,

* Also called the Arbeitsgemeinschaft für Osteosynthesefragen (AO).

and refinement that exists within the necessarily strict rules of the internal fixation method. In this way we seek to contribute to as well as to stimulate the search for rational solutions to surgical problems.

It is assumed throughout that the reader is familiar with the technical fundamentals of internal fixation, and so these details are omitted. Instead, special indications and technical refinements are presented on the basis of case examples. Because an endless variety of situations can arise in orthopedic surgery (a circumstance that is attracting more and more surgeons to the field), we have taken care that our examples can readily be applied to novel situations.

We now credit, in alphabetic order, those who contributed most to the techniques presented: R. BLATTER, A. BOITZY, C. BRUNNER, O. ĈECH, A. DEBRUNNER, F. MAGERL, G. SEGMÜLLER, G. STÜHMER, and B.G. WEBER.

We thus express thanks to those colleagues in our clinic who agreed to having their ideas published. But we are also grateful to our illustrators, H. and K. SCHUMACHER, our photographer, M. SCHAFFNER, and our chief secretary, U. OETLIKER, who contributed so much to the preparation of the manuscript. Finally, we thank Springer-Verlag for their patience with us and especially for their efficient work in bringing the book to press.

St. Gall, Fall 1981

CH.F. BRUNNER
B.G. WEBER

Contents

1 Lag Screws

The lag screw provides stability by exerting interfragmental compression.

1.1 Subchondral Placement of the Screw Head

In certain fractures, stabilization can be achieved only by applying the lag-screw principle. Occasionally, moreover, it is necessary to insert the screw from the articular surface. To permit overgrowth of the screw head with new cartilage (fibrocartilage), it is necessary that the screw head be countersunk so that it will not distrub the articular surface. This is done with a countersink, such as that for malleolar screws with a centering pin 3.2 mm in diameter. When the screw is removed at a later date, an arthrotomy must be done, and the new cartilage covering the screw head must be resected.

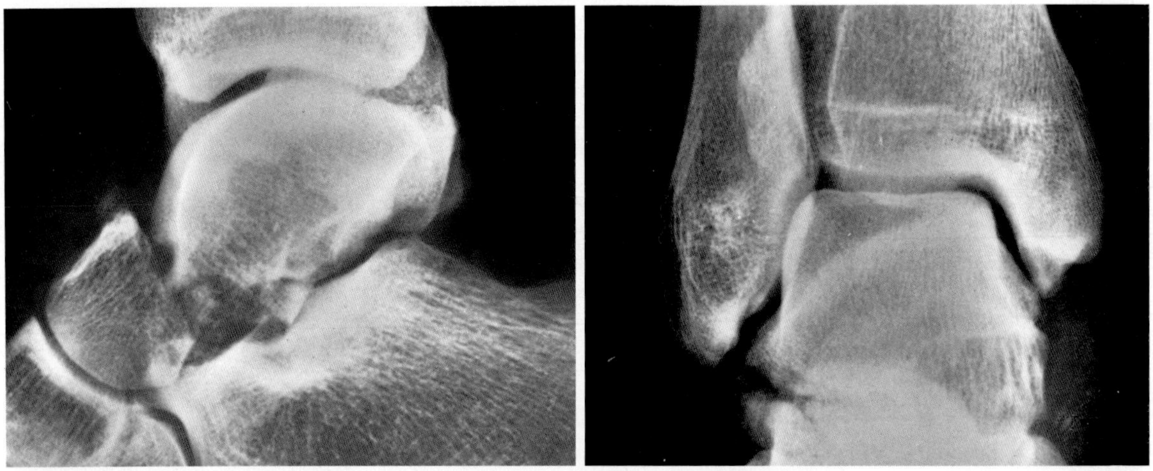

a

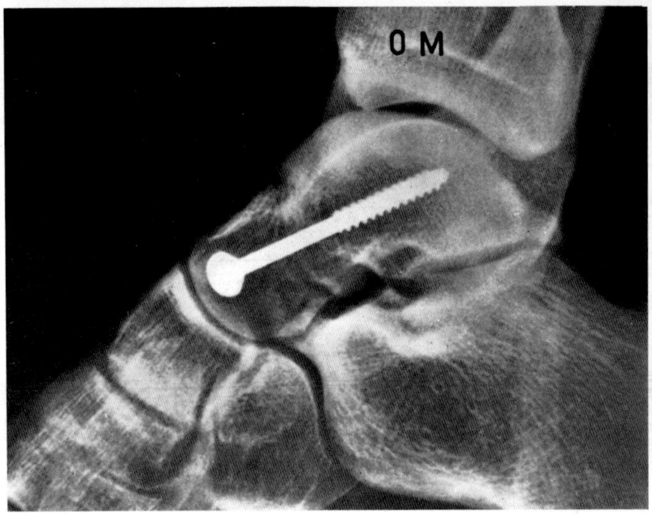

b

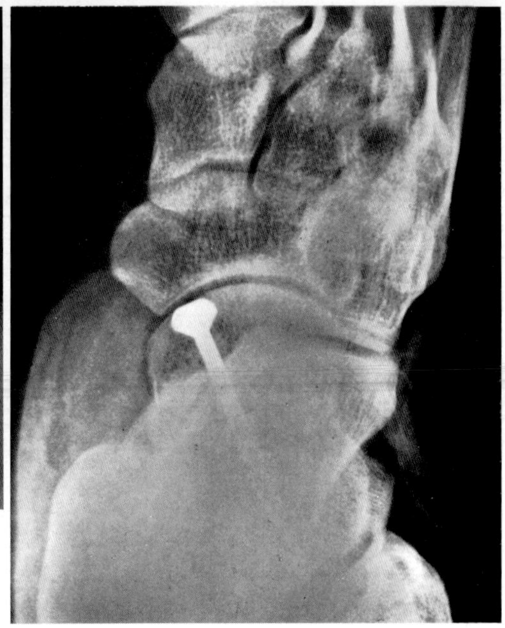

Example 1: Displaced fracture of the neck of the talus (Fig. 1)

The problem: The fracture must be anatomically reduced and stabilized. Plating is impossible, a lag screw would cross the fracture plane at too great an angle, and fixation with Kirschner wires would be unstable on exercise and would require external immobilization in plaster.

The solution: The talonavicular joint is opened from a dorsomedial approach, medial to the tendon of the anterior tibialis muscle. The fracture itself is anatomically reduced and temporarily fixed with a Kirschner wire. On plantar flexion of the foot, the head of the talus presents in the arthrotomy. A screw can now be inserted from the articular surface, crossing the fracture line at a right angle and compressing the fragments.

Important: After the gliding hole is drilled, it is countersunk so that the screw head will lie beneath the cartilage surface.

Fig. 1a–d. Subchondral placement of the screw head in a talus neck fracture. B.W., ♂, age 41, No. 134809.
a Displaced fracture of the talus neck.
b *Lag-screw fixation:* The countersunk screw head is clearly visible in the anteroposterior (AP) film.
c *Operative technique:* The proximal gliding hole is enlarged with the countersink to allow subchondral placement of the screw head.
d *Four and a half months after operation:* Fracture healed, talonavicular joint normal

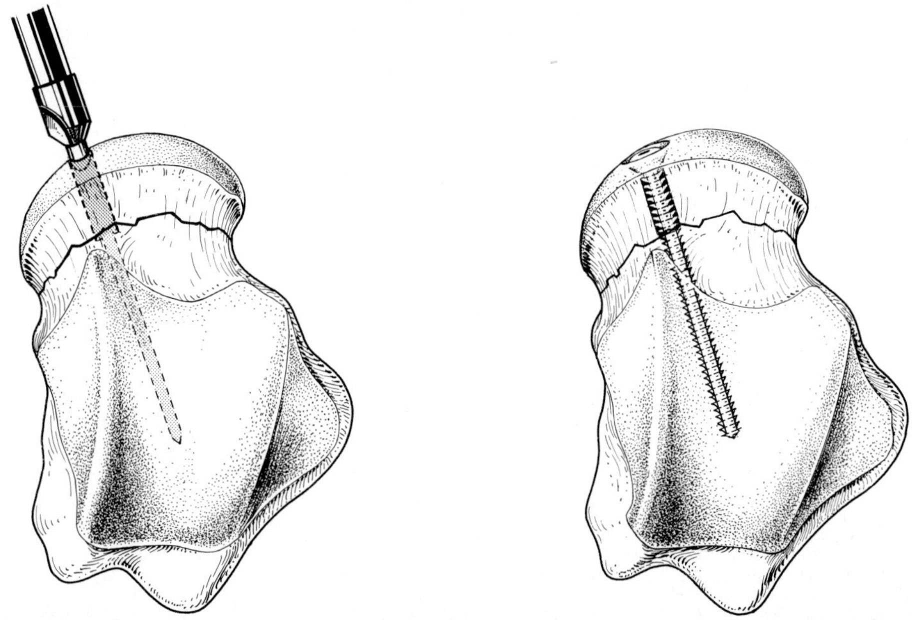

c

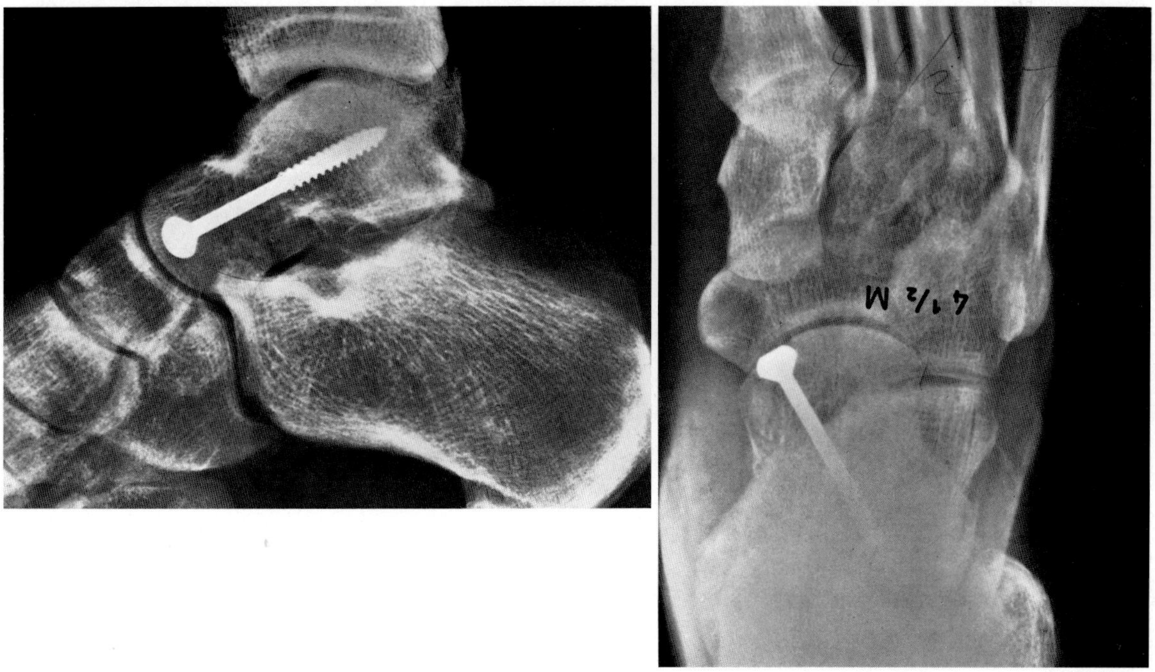

d

Example 2: Pseudarthrosis following a distal metacarpal fracture (Fig. 2)

The problem: The distal fragment is too small to allow secure plating of the fracture. How can the small and now porotic fragment be stably fixed?

The solution: Arthrotomy of the metacarpophalangeal joint and axial screw fixation of the pseudarthrosis will achieve this. The screw head is countersunk below the cartilage surface.

Fig. 2a–c. Subchondral placement of the screw head in subcapital pseudarthrosis of the fifth metacarpal.
K.L., ♂, age 40, No. 112179.
a Unstable internal fixation, pseudarthrosis.
b *Axial screw fixation:* The head of the lag screw is countersunk below the cartilage surface.
c *Three and a half years after screw fixation:* Pseudarthrosis healed, no signs of arthrosis of the metacarpophalangeal joint

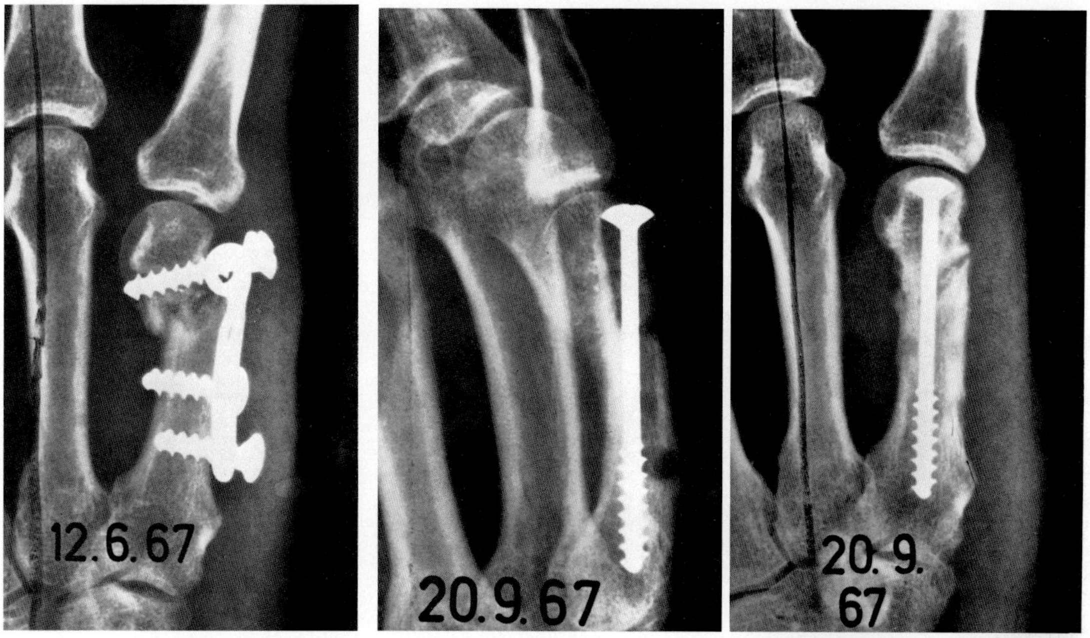

a, b

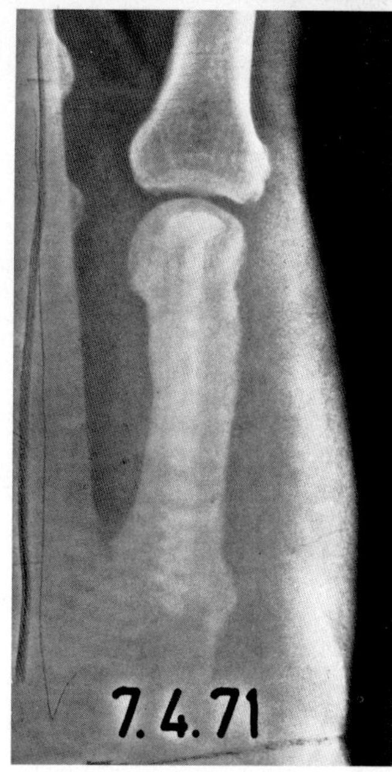

c

a
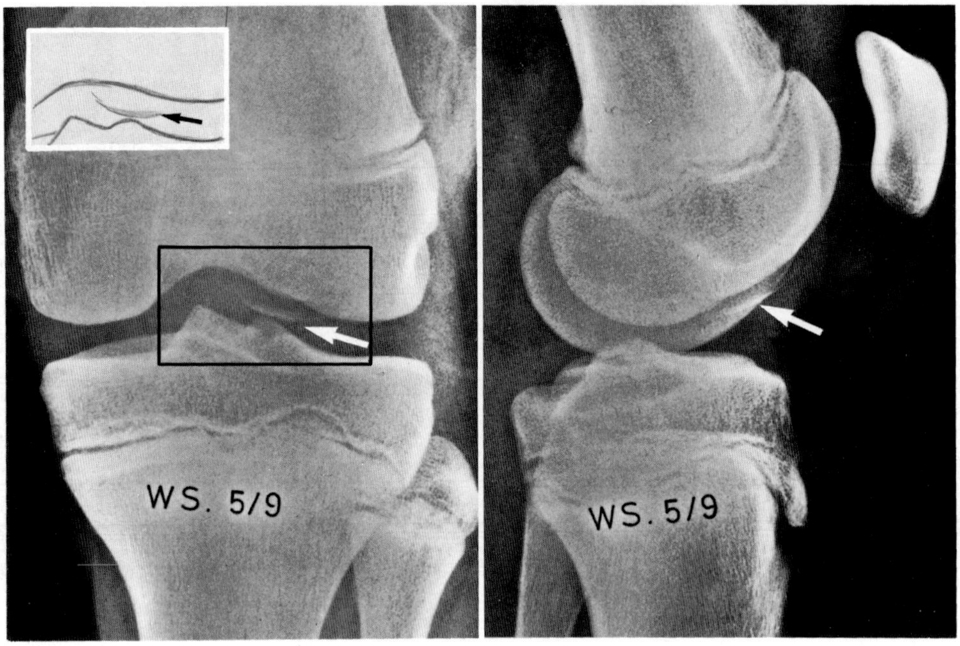

Example 3: Osteochondral fracture of the femoral condyle (Fig. 3)

The problem: A lag screw inserted from the metaphysis would penetrate and damage the epiphyseal plate. The articular fragment would also be too small and thin to be satisfactorily engaged by the screw thread.

The solution: After arthrotomy, the screw is inserted from the articular surface without damaging the epiphyseal plate. The screw heads are countersunk below the cartilage surface.

Fig. 3a–c. Countersunk screw for osteochondral fracture of the femoral condyle in an adolescent.
S.A., ♂, age 15, no. 166842.
a Osteochondral fragment is faintly visible (*arrow*).
b *Arthrotomy and screw fixation:* The screw heads project into the joint space, but they are countersunk in the cartilage.
c *One year after injury:* Fracture healed, no joint derangement

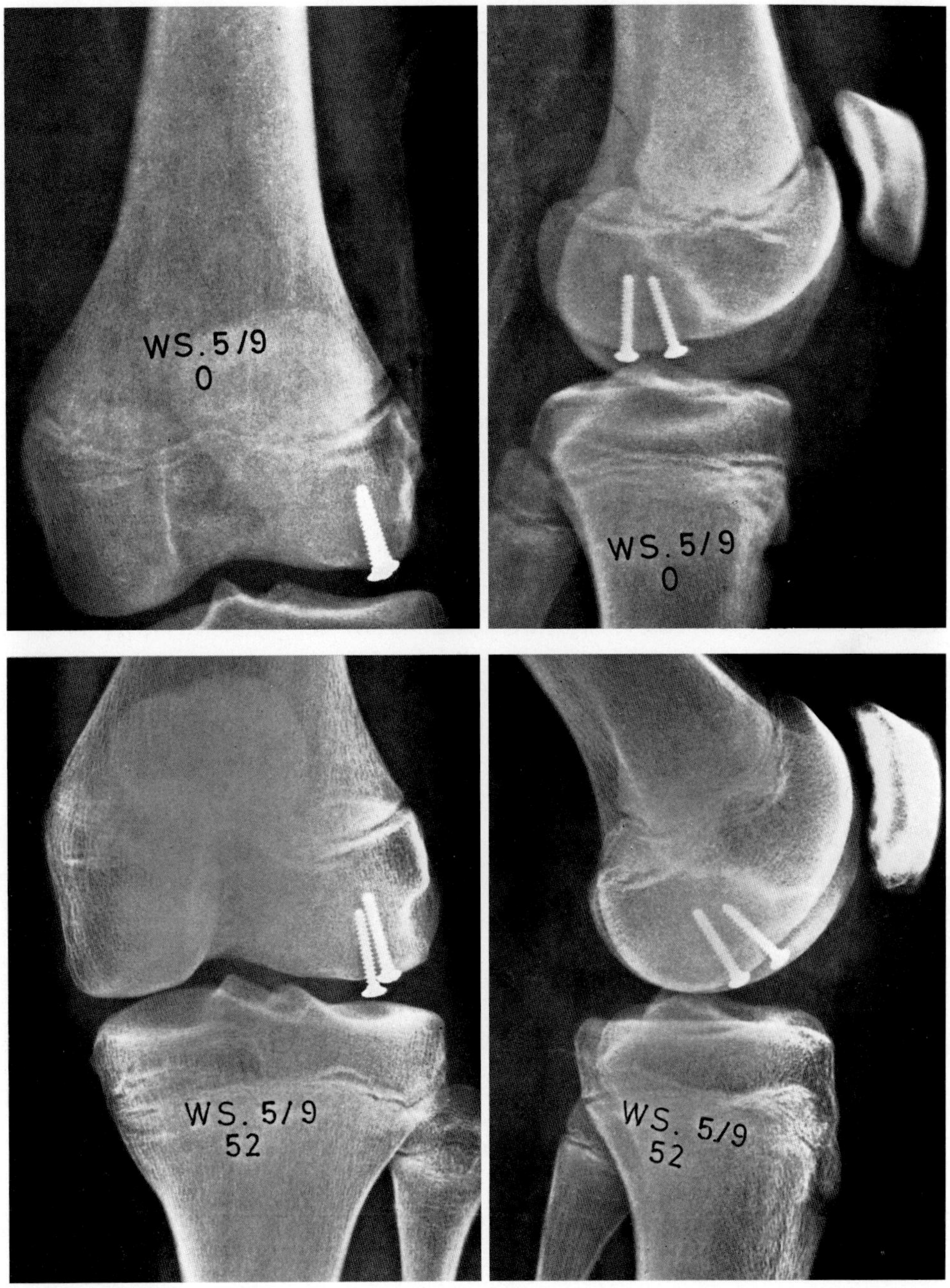

b

c

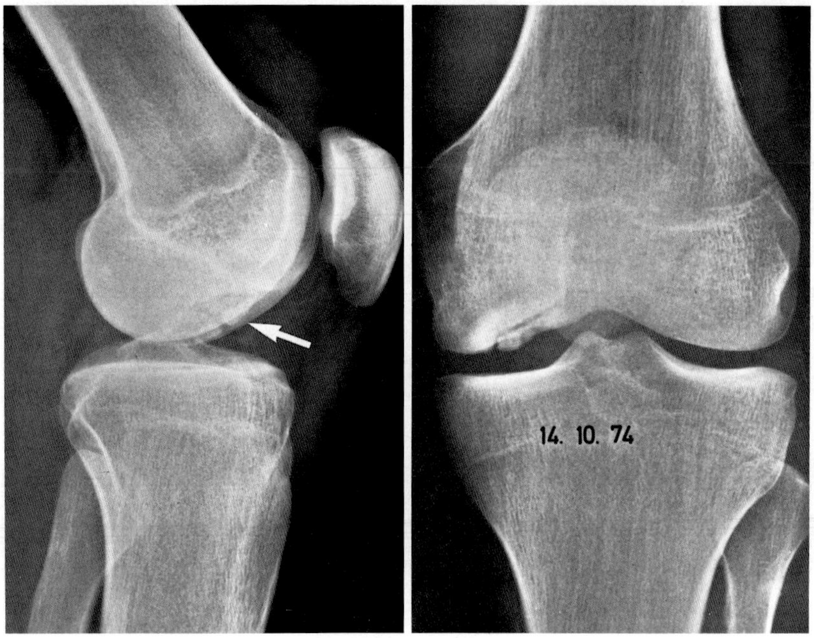

a

Example 4: Osteochondritis dissecans of the femoral condyle (Fig. 4)

The problem: The osteochondritic fragment can be revascularized from the femoral condyle only under absolutely stable conditions.

The solution: Following arthrotomy, the fragment is removed, its cavity is freshened, and several holes are drilled through the sclerotic zone. Then the fragment is replaced in its cavity and fixed with lag screws.

Fig. 4a–c. Screw insertion from the joint surface in osteochondritis dissecans.
L.J., ♂, age 19, No. 181543.
a Osteochondritic fragment with sclerosis of the underlying bone.
b *Arthrotomy:* The fragment is removed from its cavity, and the sclerotic bone is perforated with multiple 2-mm drill holes to promote revascularization. Then the fragment is replaced in its cavity and fixed with two small lag screws, which are countersunk below the cartilage surface.
c *Fifteen months after operation:* Owing to the stable fixation, the fragment has become revascularized and is well incorporated

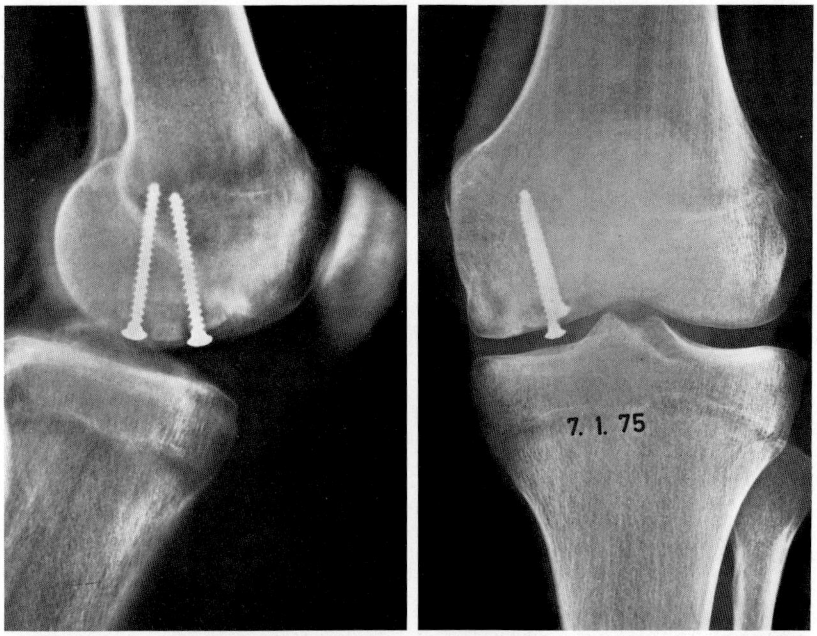

b

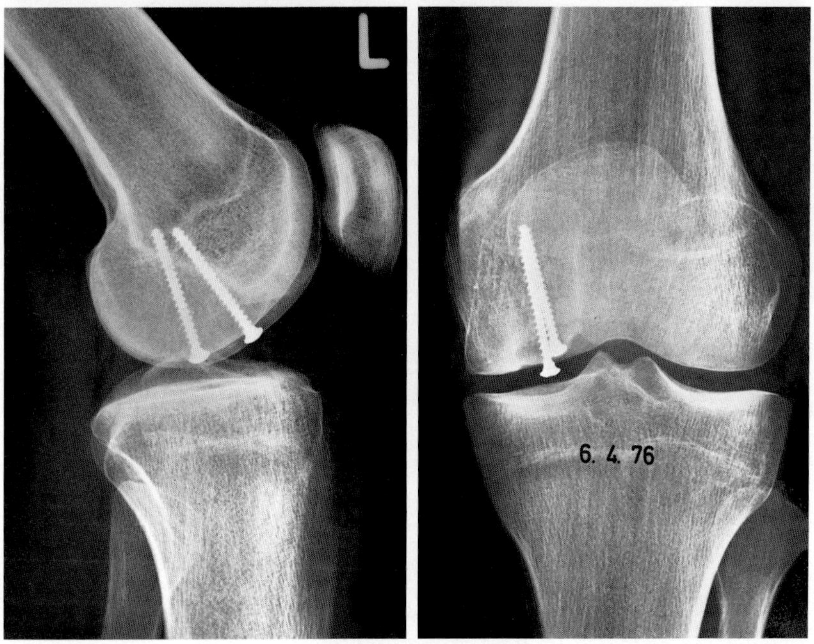

c

Example 5: "Chisel" fracture of the head of the radius (Fig. 5)

The problem: An internal fixation can be carried out only from the articular surface.

The solution: Kocher's approach is used. Damage to the proximal radioulnar joint is avoided by subchondral countersinking of the screw head. Lag-screw fixation allows early mobilization.

Fig. 5a–c. Screw fixation of a chisel fracture of the radial head.
H.M., ♂, age 21, No. 51351.
a Intra-articular fracture with step.
b *Operation:* Anatomic reduction, fracture stabilization with lag screw, subchondral placement of screw head. Postoperative mobilization.
c *Five months after injury:* Functional and anatomic healing

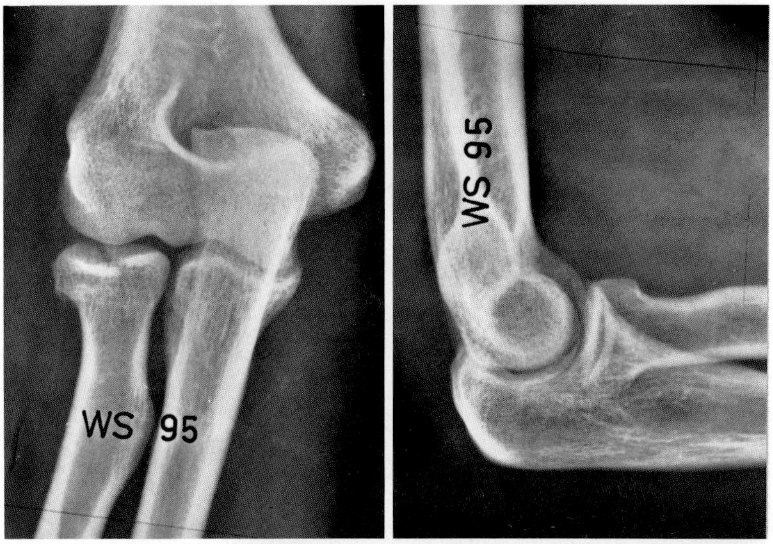

a

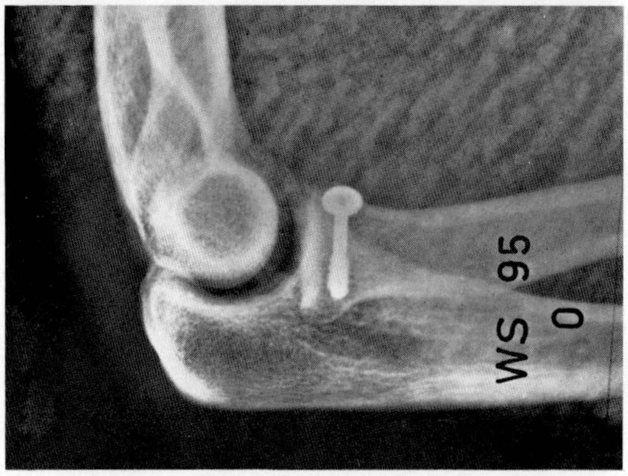

b

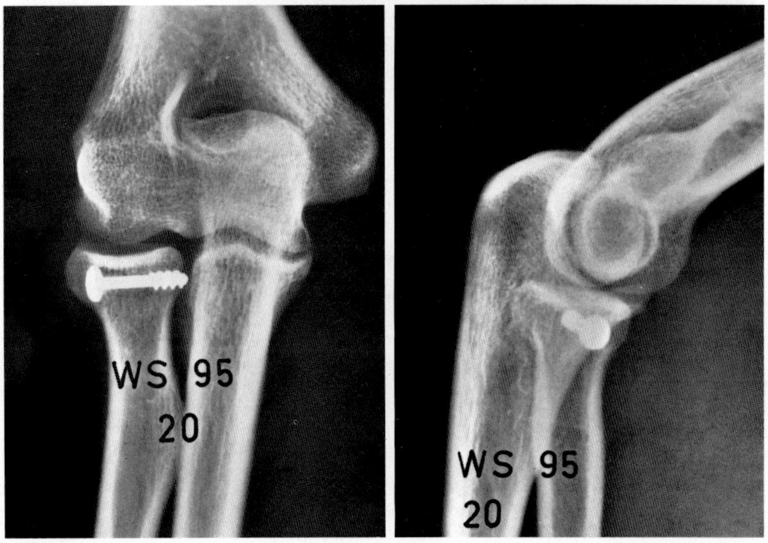

c

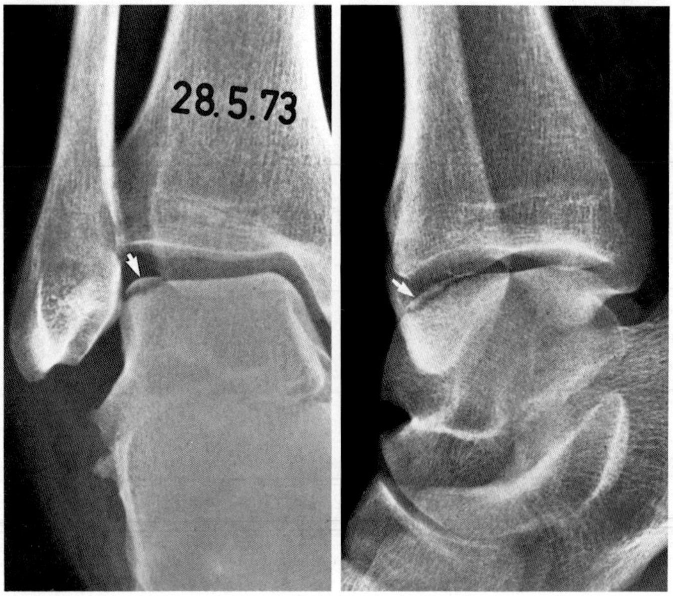

a

Example 6: Fracture of the border of the talar dome (Fig. 6)

The problem: An internal fixation can be carried out only from the articular surface.

The solution: Anterolateral arthrotomy of the ankle joint. The fragment is demonstrated by maximum plantar flexion of the foot, so that the screw can be correctly inserted. An analogous procedure is used in osteochondritis dissecans of the lateral or medial talar dome. Osteotomy of one malleolus is sometimes necessary for adequate exposure.

Fig. 6a–d. Screw fixation of a marginal fracture of the talar dome.
O.T., ♀, age 24, No. 168272.
a *Postinjury roentgenogram:* Supination trauma with rupture of the collateral fibular ligaments; the marginal talus fragment has been sheared off by the fibular joint surface.
b *Operative technique:* Maximum plantar flexion allows vision into the fracture. Anatomic reduction, fixation with countersunk lag screw.
c *Reconstruction:* The space between the screw head and articular surface is filled with fibrocartilage to restore the smooth surface.
d *One year after injury:* Fragment incorporated, no signs of arthrosis

b

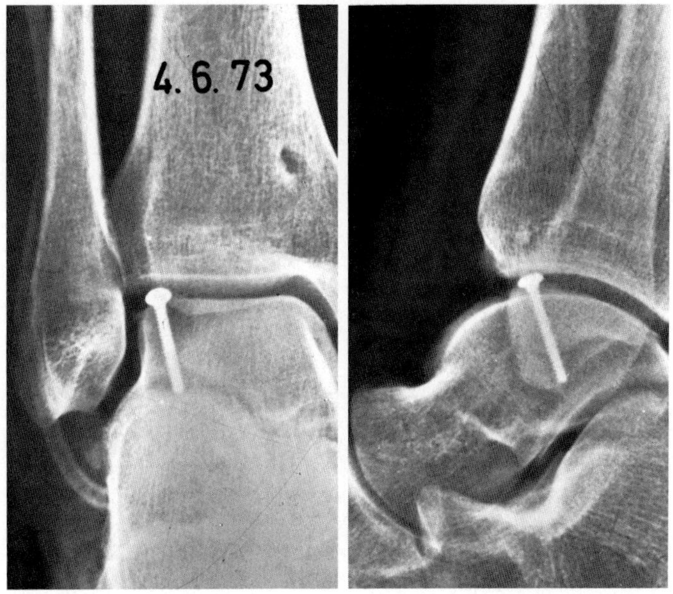

c

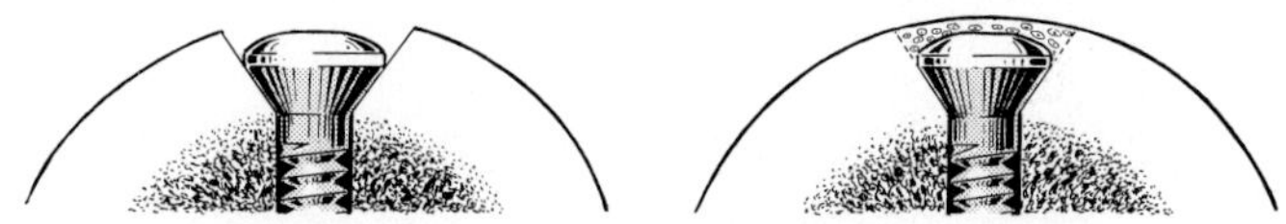

d

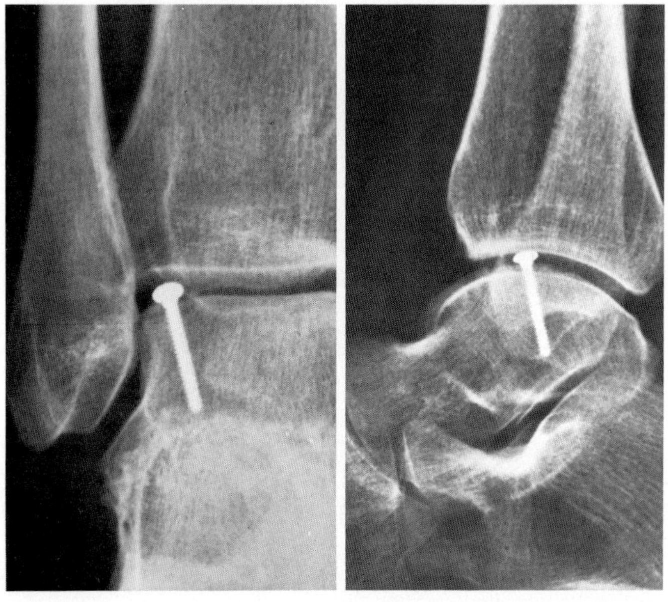

Example 7: Dislocation of the femoral head with a tangential chip fracture (Fig. 7)

The problem: Following closed reduction, the shearing fracture must be managed through an anterior hip arthrotomy. Without treatment, the congruity of the hip joint would be lost.

The solution: In the same way that material is attached to a chair with closely spaced upholstery nails, the osteochondral fragments are tacked down to the femoral head with small lag screws; again, the screw heads are subchondrally placed.

Fig. 7a–d. Screw fixation of chip fragments in a fracture-dislocation of the femoral head.
H.A., ♂, age 15, No. 168940.
a *Obturator dislocation:* Cap-shaped osteochondral fragments, still attached to the synovial reflection.
b Fixation with lag screws countersunk below the cartilage surface.
c Just as material is attached to a chair with closely spaced upholstery nails, the chip fragments and synovial reflection are fixed to the femoral head with small lag screws.
d *Two years and 10 months after injury:* Normal joint congruity

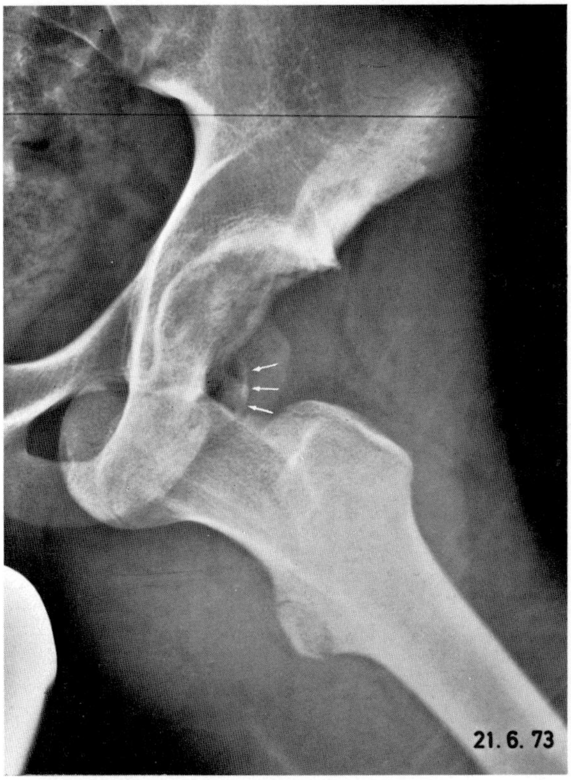

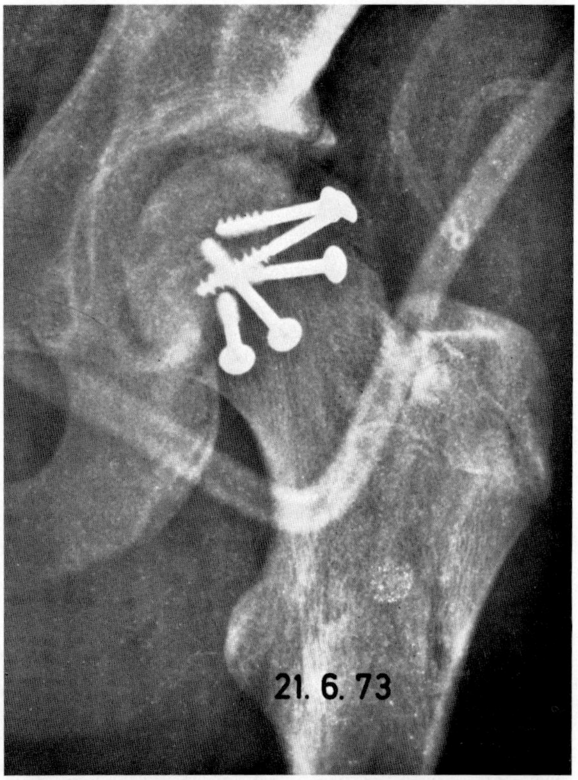

a, b

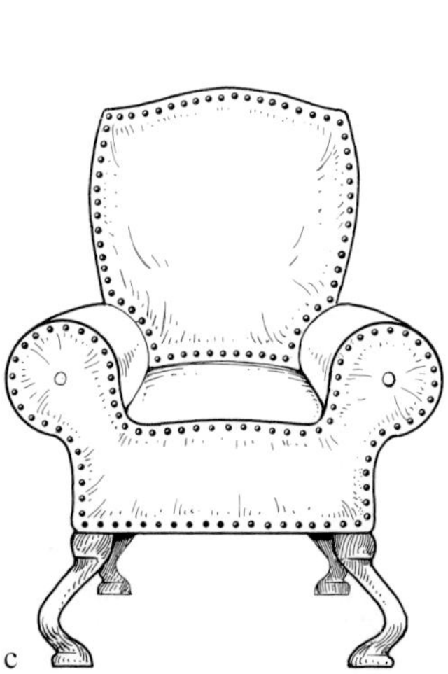

c

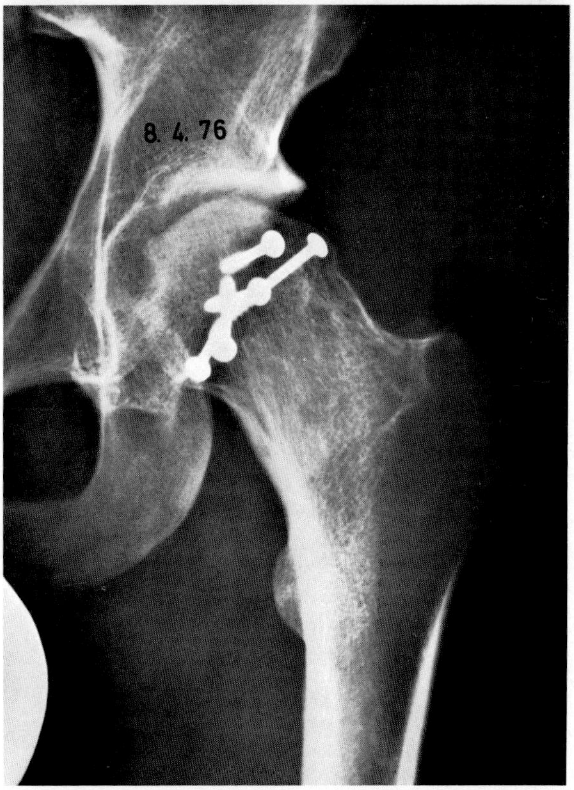

d

1.2 Lag Screws in Tendon Insertion

In the internal fixation of avulsion fractures, care must be taken to avoid damaging the tendinous or ligamentous fibers that radiate into the fragment. Very small avulsion fragments can be managed with a transosseous suture. For larger fragments of tendon insertions, screw fixation is advised. The screw head damages only a few tendinous fibers, and the resulting stability allows postoperative mobilization.

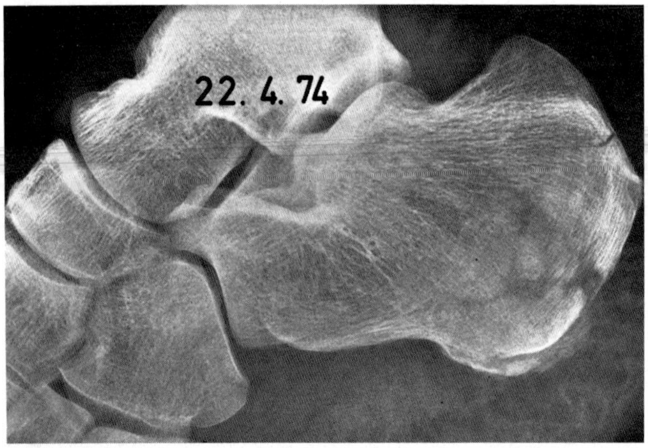

a

Example 1: "Duckbill" fracture of the calcaneus (Fig. 8)

The problem: Besides instability of the tendon insertion, there is an incongruity of the subtalar joint in this type of fracture, since the displaced avulsion fragment forms part of the articular surface of the posterior talocalcanean joint. Thus, internal fixation must have two aims: to restore the tension resistance of the Achilles tendon and to reestablish the congruity of the subtalar joint.

The solution: A stab incision is made through the Achilles tendon, followed by closed drilling and screw insertion under image intensifier control. With successful fixation of the fragment, the congruity of the joint surfaces is automatically restored.

Fig. 8a–d. Screw fixation of a longitudinal (duckbill) fracture of the calcaneus. D.V., ♂, age 33, No. 76867.
a *Calcaneus fracture:* The avulsion fragment is displaced in a cephalad direction by the pull of the Achilles tendon; the subtalar joint is incongruent.
b *Principle of treatment:* The "bill" is held shut with a lag screw.
c *Operation:* The fracture is reduced and fixed with a lag screw, and the congruity of the subtalar joint is reestablished.
d *One year after injury:* Complete healing with no complications

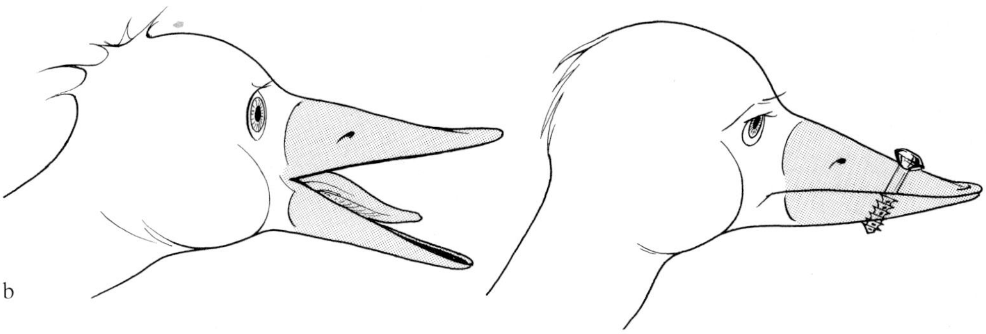

b

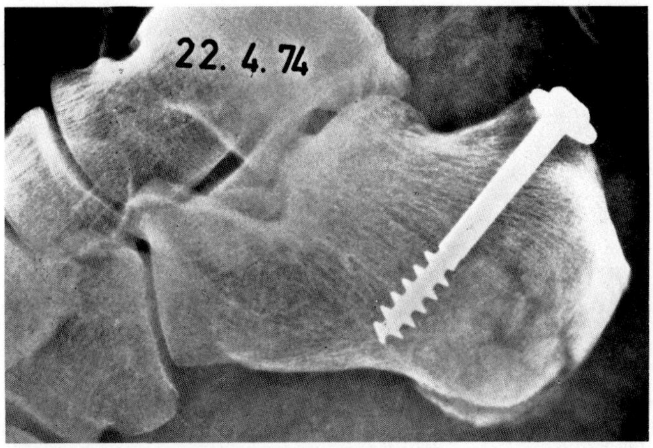

c

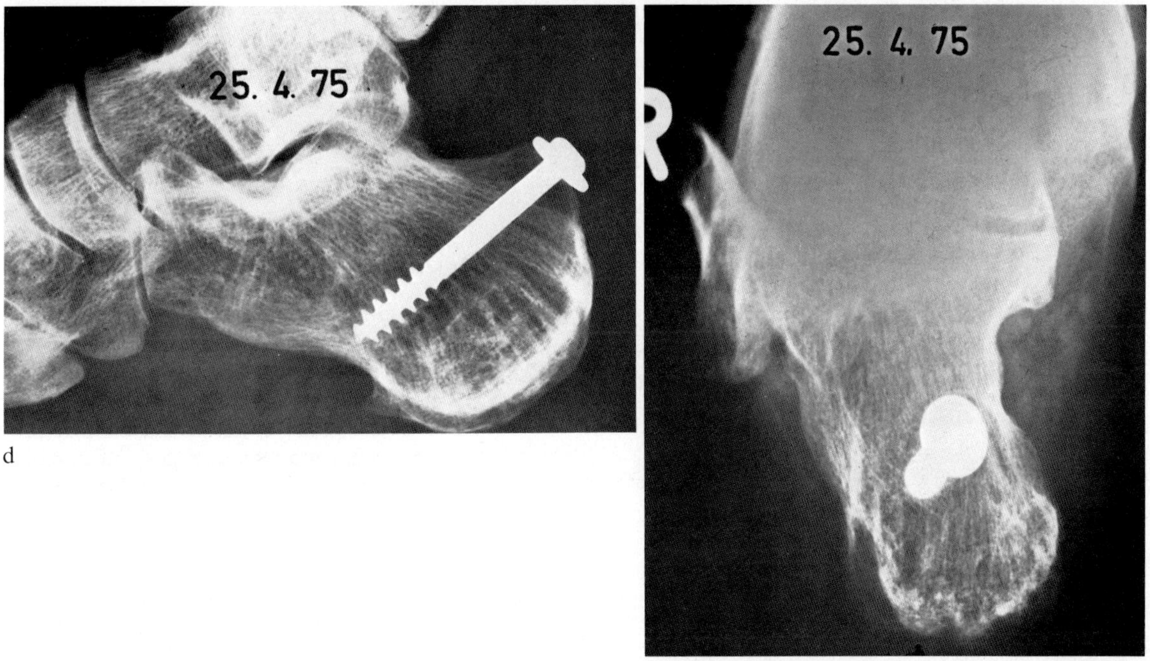

d

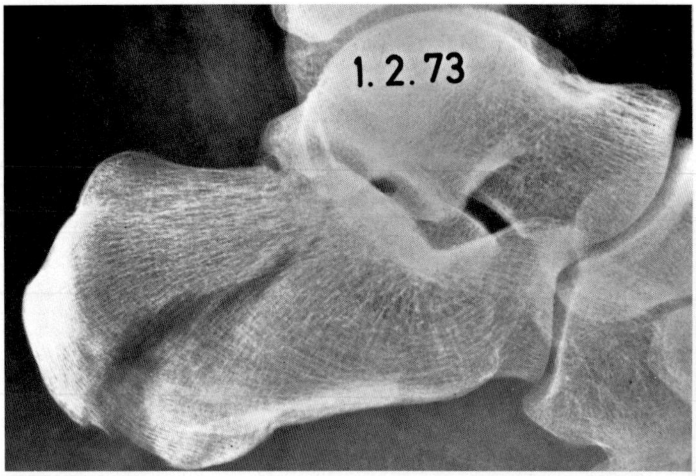

a

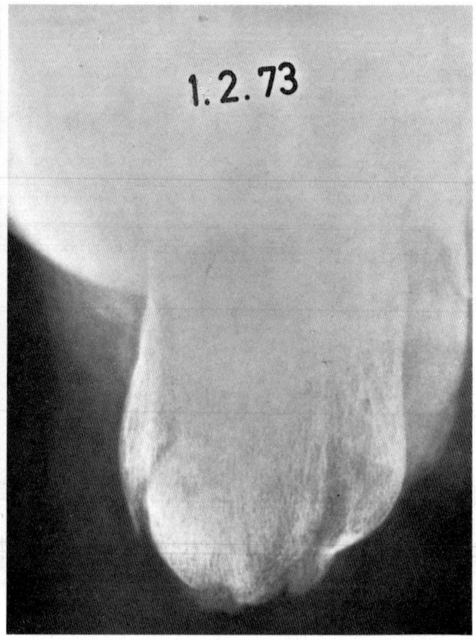

Example 2: Duckbill fracture of the calcaneus with associated sagittal fracture of the distal fragment (Fig. 9)

The problem: The screw thread can engage the plantar surface of the calcaneus only after the stable screw fixation of the sagittal fracture.

The solution: The fracture is carefully exposed from a lateral approach; this is followed by gradual reduction and screw fixation of the two fracture components.

Fig. 9a–d. Multidimensional screw fixation of a duckbill fracture of the calcaneus with an additional fracture line. G.F., ♂, age 28, No. 141195.
a *Calcaneus fracture:* Broadly open duckbill with associated sagittal fractures.
b Open crocodile jaws remain closed when pressed together by an external force.
c *Internal fixation by this principle:* The fractures are reduced from a lateral approach, and transverse screw fixation of both lateral surfaces of the calcaneus (the "lower jaw") follows. Then a lag screw is driven in through a stab incicion from the Achilles tendon insertion.
d *Two years and 4 months after injury:* Excellent end-result

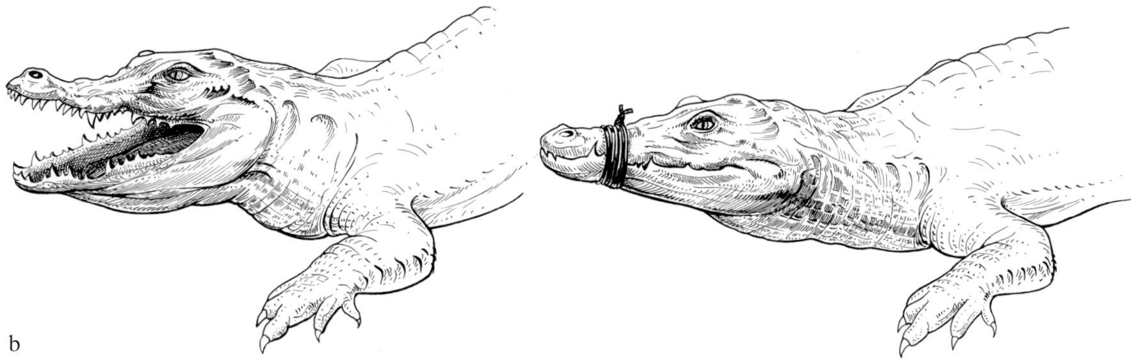

b

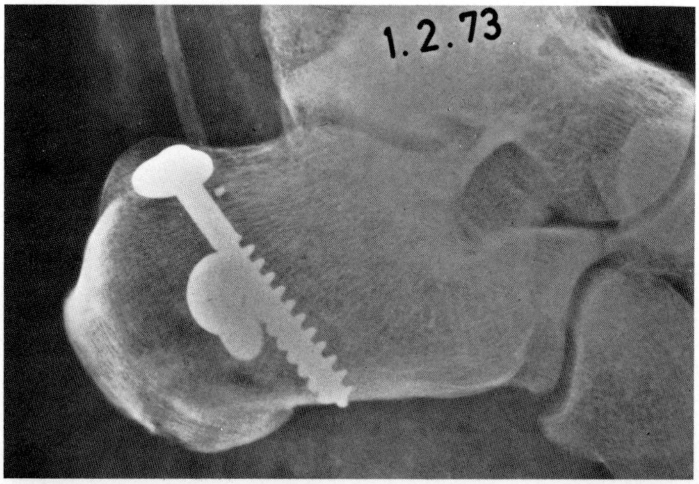

c

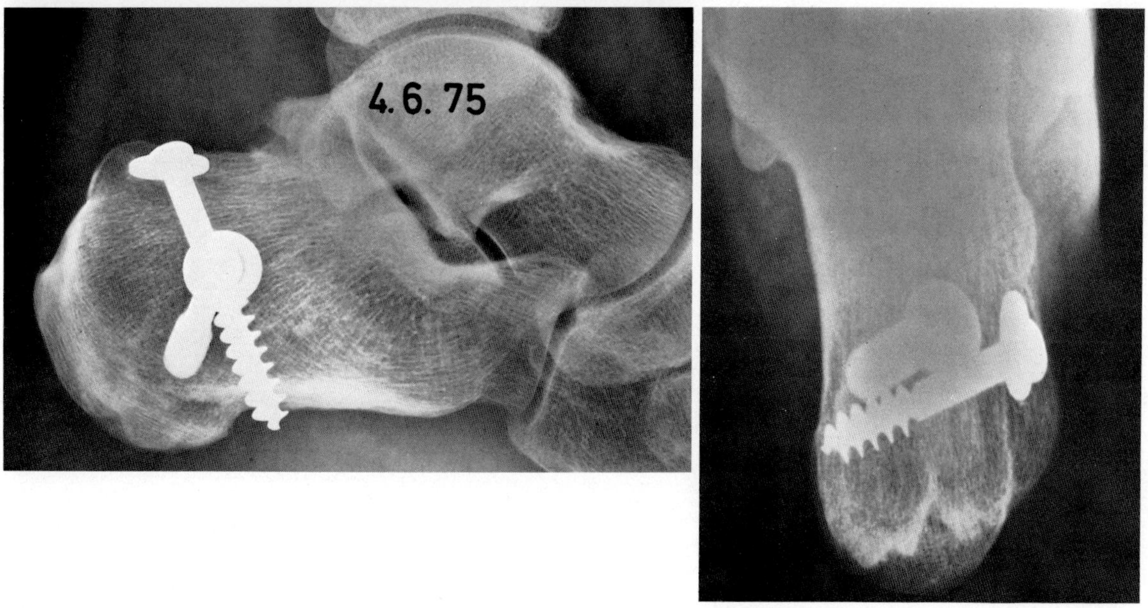

d

Example 3: Polar avulsion fracture of the patella (Fig. 10)

The problem: The avulsion fragment is too small for tension band wiring.

The solution: The patellar ligament is split longitudinally, and a lag screw is inserted through the apex of the patella.

Fig. 10a–d. Screw fixation of a caudal pole avulsion fracture of the patella. D.A., ♀, age 21, No. 194681.
a Distal pole avulsion.
b *Technique:* A transverse skin incision is made, and the patellar tendon is split longitudinally. The fracture is manually reduced, the gliding hole and thread hole are drilled, and a small cortical lag screw is inserted.
c Postoperative position of screw.
d *One year after injury:* Complete recovery

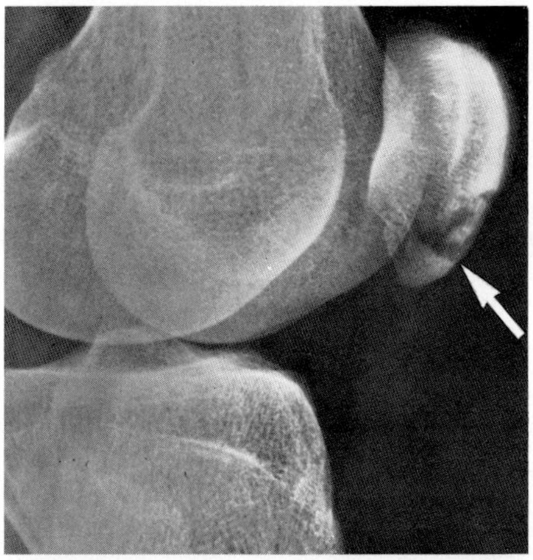

a

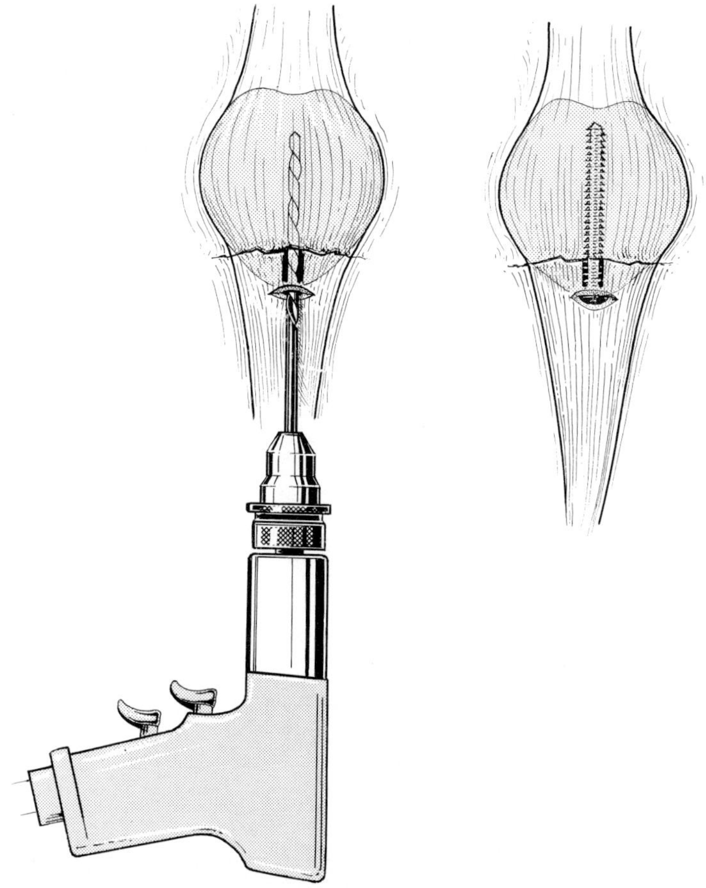

b

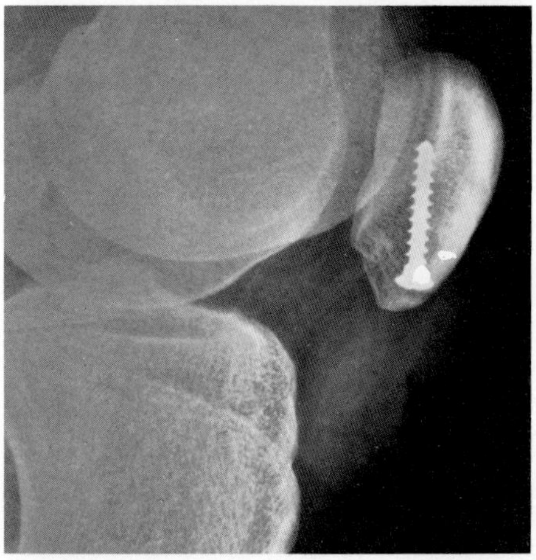

c

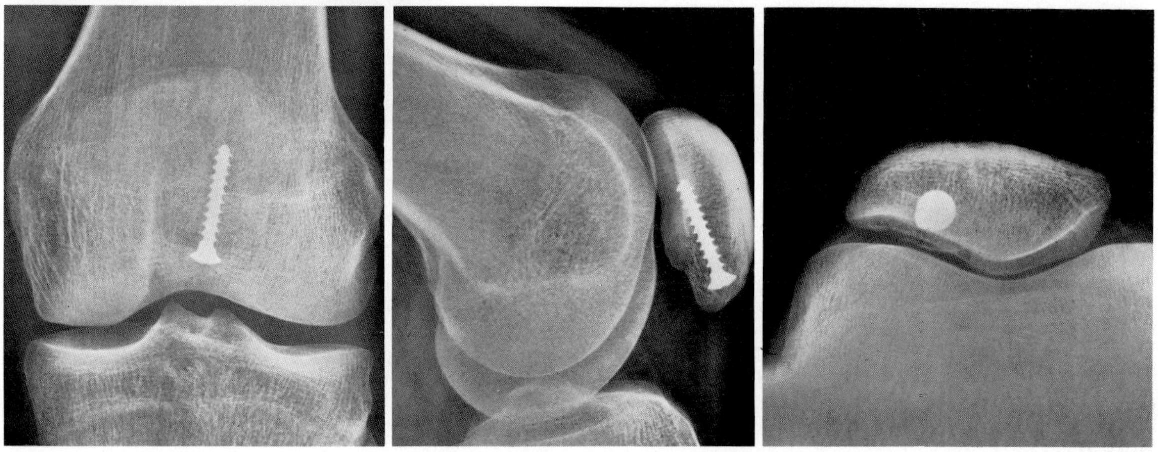

d

1.3 Internal Screw Fixation of the Vertebral Column

Lag screws may be used in spinal fusions to help reduce the danger of pseudarthrosis.

Example 1: Screw fixation of the pars interarticularis in spondylolysis (Fig. 11)

With the slightest degree of slip, it is assumed that the intervertebral disc is undamaged. A normal state can then be restored with bony union of the pedicles.

The problem: In bilateral spondylolysis of the pars interarticularis, there must be absolute mechanical rest between the fragments before bony union can occur.

The solution: From a posterior approach, the pars interarticularis is fixed bilaterally with screws to promote bony union.

Fig. 11 a, b. Screw fixation of the pars interarticularis in spondylolysis.
M.M., ♀, age 34, No. 222165.
a Spondylolysis of L-5 with chronic low back pain.
b *Screw fixation of the pars interarticularis:* Both screws stabilize the bony defect, thus enabling the spondylolysis to heal after a small cancellous graft is applied. The screws are passed from the caudal articular process through the defect toward the pedicles, or directly into the cranial articular process

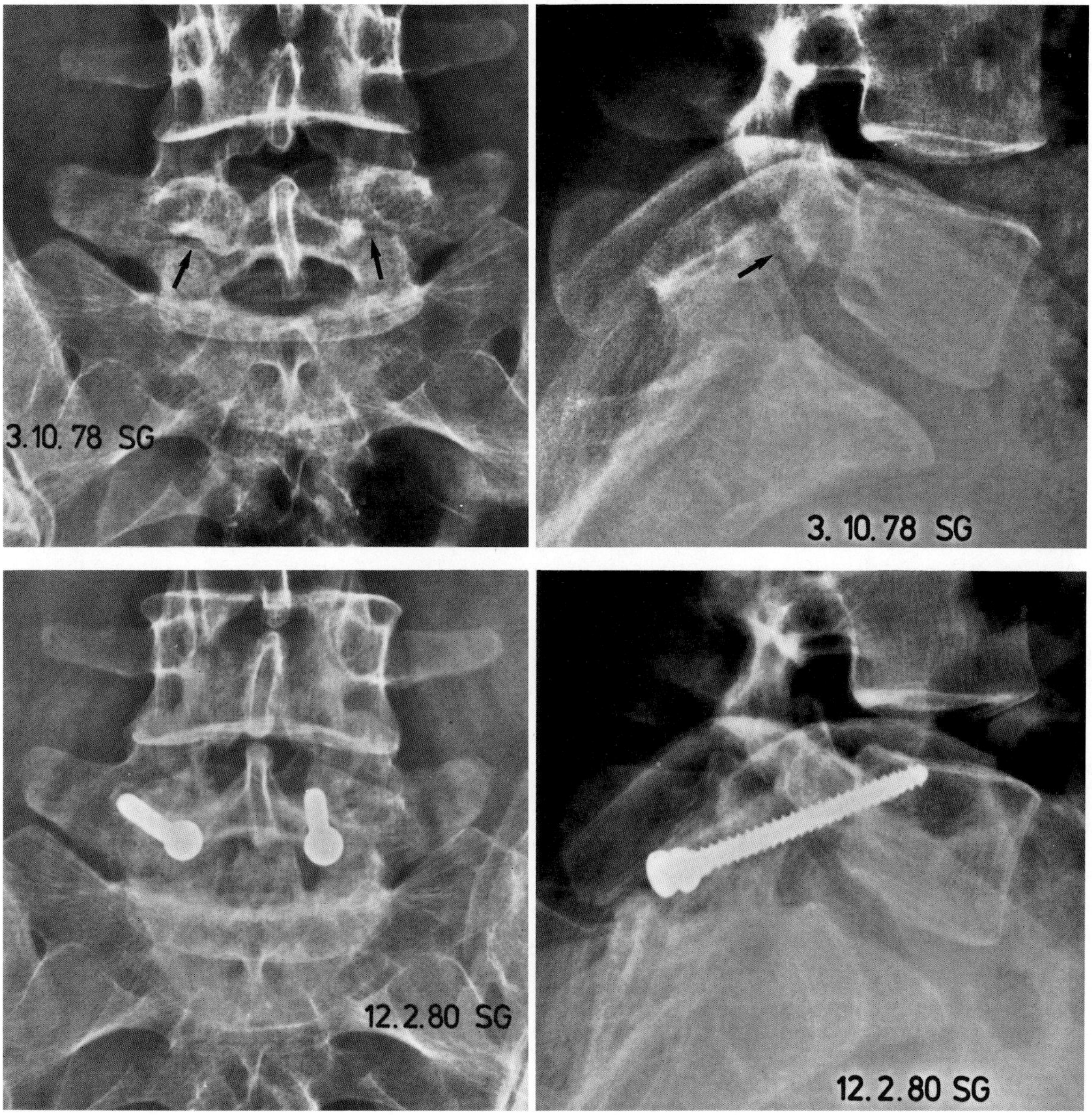

a

b

Example 2: Screw fixation of the pars interarticularis in interbody fusion for spondylolisthesis (Fig. 12)

With a high-grade slip, the pelvis is malaligned, and lumbosacral stability is impaired. Reduction of the slip is therefore desirable. This reduction is best accomplished by an anterior interbody graft fusion with the aid of Hohmann retractors.

The problem: Maintenance of the reduction is hampered by the propensity to slip caused by a lack of "tethering" by the vertebral arch. As a result, the interbody fusion is subjected to shearing forces which interfere with incorporation and vascularization of the bone grafts and predispose to pseudarthrosis.

The solution: In a second operation, the screw fixation of the pars interarticularis and screw arthrodesis of the facet joints is undertaken from a posterior approach. The tethering function of the vertebral arch is restored. Bony union of the interbody fusion is no longer hampered by shearing forces.

Fig. 12a–c. Posterior reinforcement of an interbody spinal fusion.
R. B., ♂, age 40, No. 209035.
a Spondylolisthesis of L-4–L-5 with spondylolysis and root irritation.
b *Anterior fusion:* Optimum reduction and interbody fusion with corticocancellous iliac grafts. Two weeks later, through a posterior approach, the spondylolysis and deformed facet joints are fixed with lag screws; this is followed by a posterior fusion.
c *Five months after operation:* Problem-free incorporation of bone grafts; anterior and posterior fusions are solid

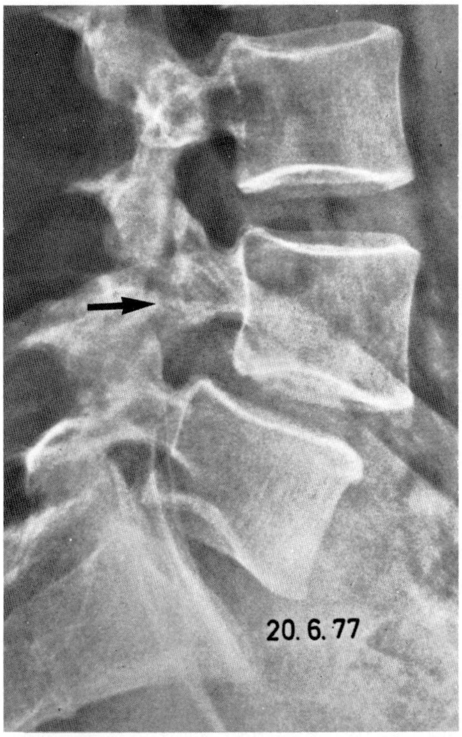

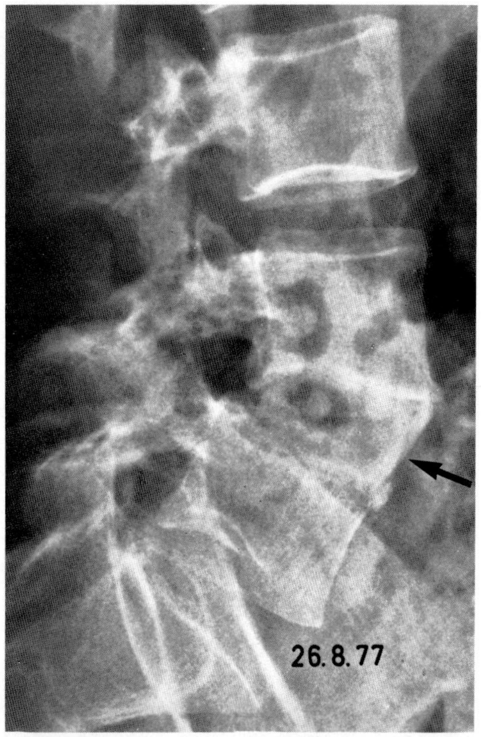

a, b

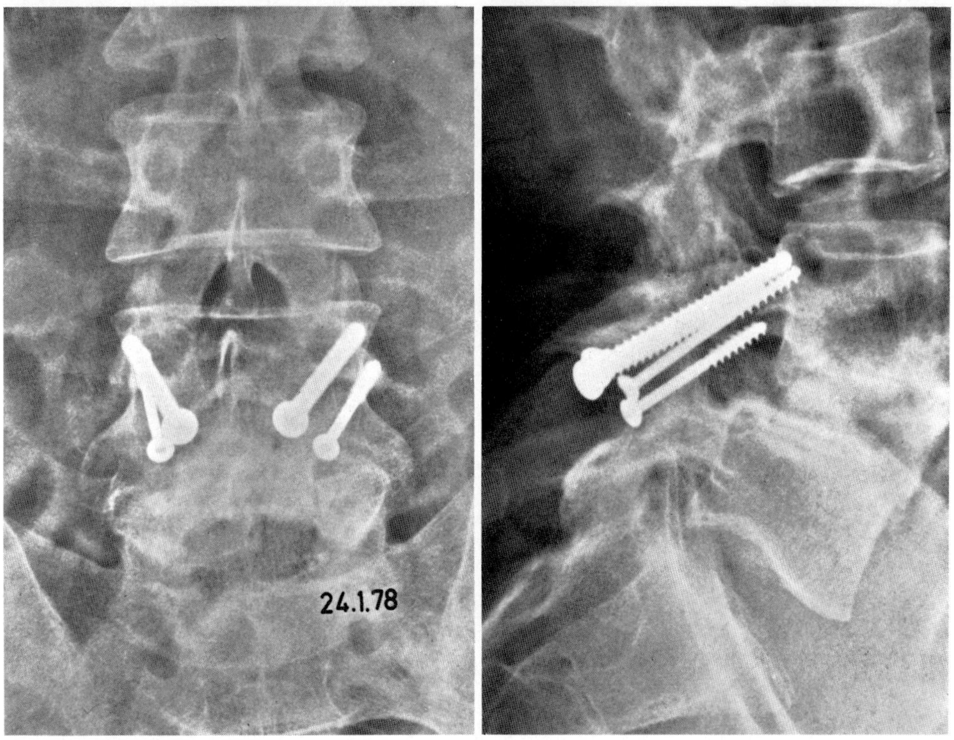

c

Example 3: Direct screw fixation of the interbody fusion (Fig. 13)

With an unstable lumbosacral junction, the placement of corticocancellous grafts may be insufficient in itself to ensure undisturbed bony union. To permit early mobilization therefore, the grafting should be augmented by compressive internal fixation.

The problem: After resection of the upper plates and placement of the grafts, there is a tendency for anterior gaping to occur even with moderate extension.

The solution: The fifth lumbar vertebral body is stabilized against the sacrum with an axial lag screw, and the anterior gape is neutralized. Owing to the mechanical rest achieved, the bone grafts are incorporated without interference.

Fig. 13a–c. Screw fixation of an interbody bone-graft fusion.
H. G., ♀, age 39, No. 208025.
a Osteochondrosis of L-5–S-1 with narrowing of disc.
b *Postoperatively:* The resected intervertebral disc is replaced with corticocancellous iliac grafts. Interbody lag-screw fixation.
c *One year after operation:* Fusion consolidated

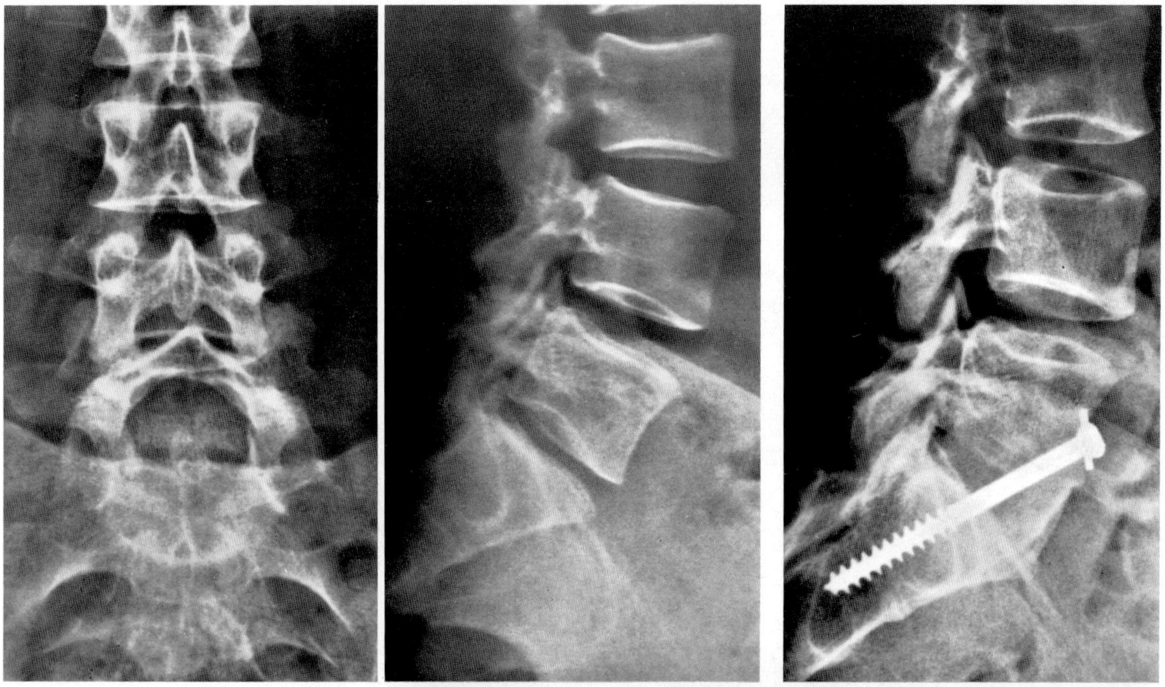

a, b

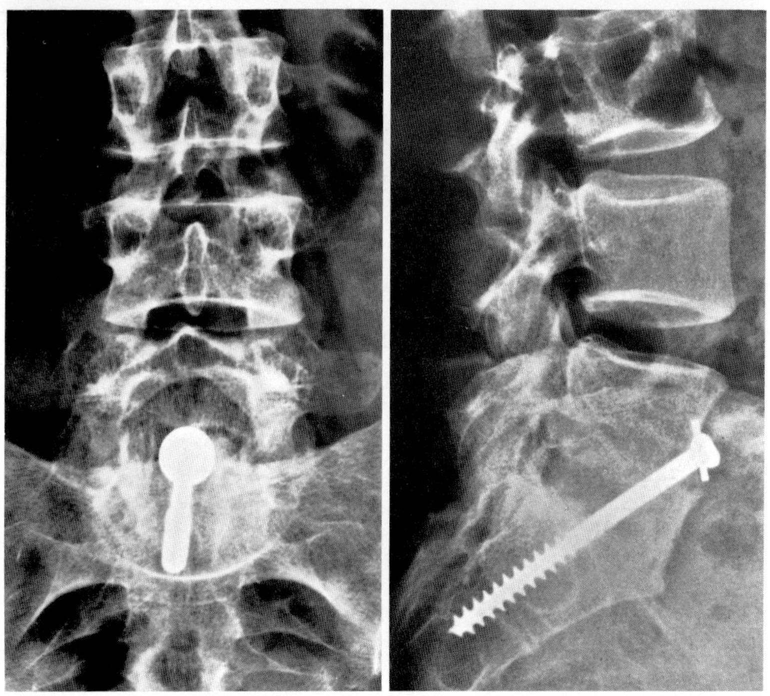

c

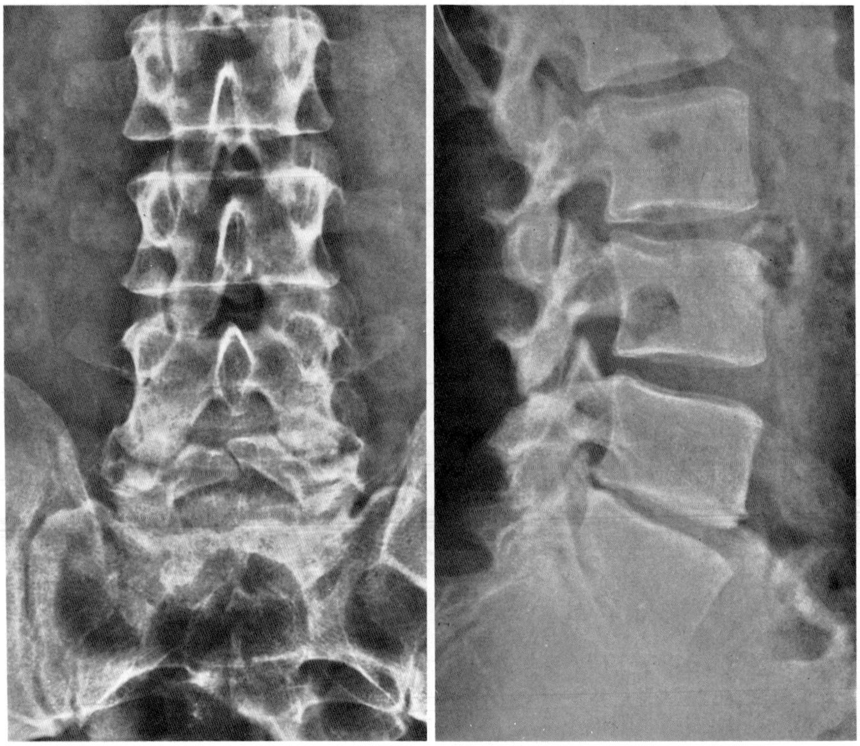

a

Example 4: "Cross-screw" fixation of the facet joints (Fig. 14)

Often it is advantageous in posterior fusions to insert screws through the facet joints after cartilage removal. This greatly enhances stability, ensuring a solid interspinous, interlaminar, and intertransverse fusion despite early mobilization.

The problem: In the lumbar region the articular surfaces are inclined in such a way that direct screw fixation is not always possible.

The solution: With cross-screw fixation, optimum compression can be exerted perpendicular to the articular surfaces. In this way stability is vastly improved. The screw holes are drilled through the spinous process, and correspondingly long screws are used.

Fig. 14a–c. Cross-screw fixation of the facet joints in a posterior fusion. B. K., ♂, age 44, No. 213918.
a Osteochondrosis of L-4–L-5–S-1.
b *One year after operation:* The crossed-screw fixation of the facet joints across the midline stabilizes the facets, allowing the posterior fusion to consolidate without interference despite early mobilization and without a plaster jacket.
c The oblique films demonstrate the extension of the screws beyond the facets.

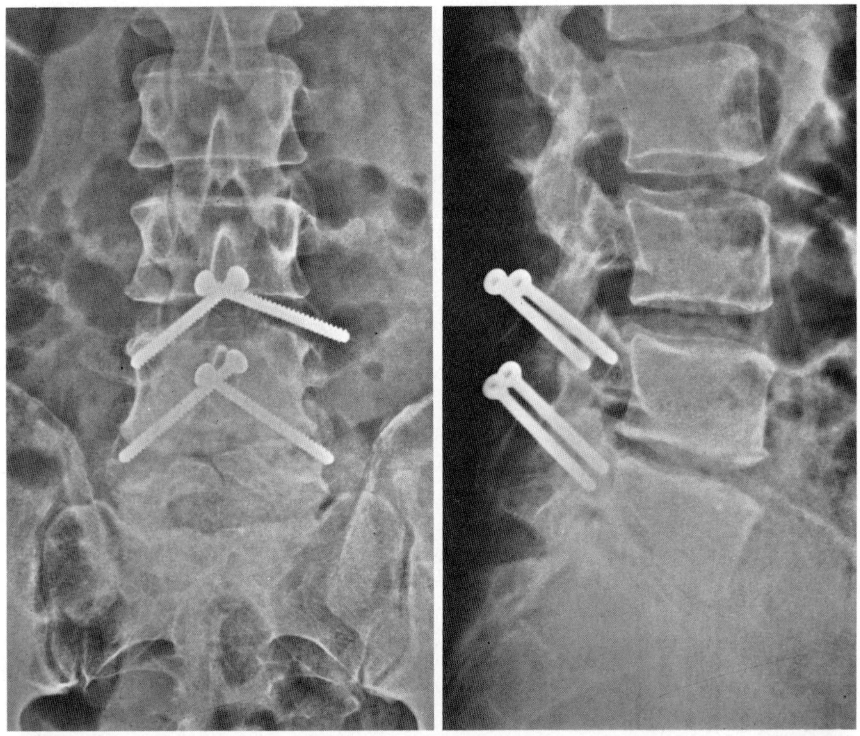

b

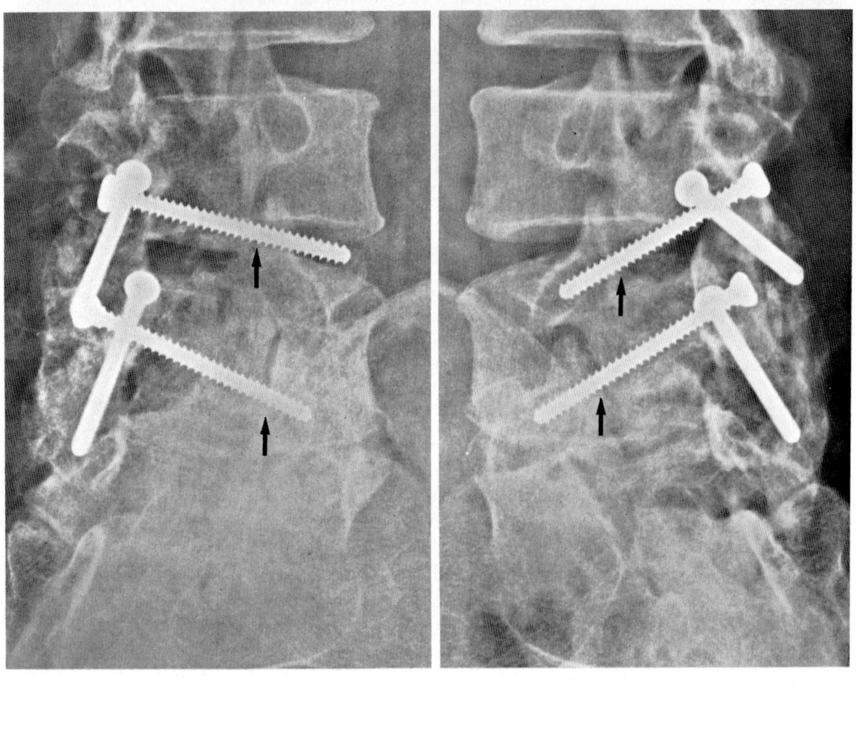

c

1.4 Screws Placed in Unusual Sites

The following examples illustrate the principle of achieving maximum strength using a minimum of fixative material, i.e., screws alone. For this purpose, it sometimes becomes necessary to insert screws in unusual locations.

Example 1: Fracture of the shoulder joint in the multiple injury patient (Fig. 15)

In this comminuted fracture, the caudal half of the glenoid cavity is displaced downward, together with a large scapular fragment.

The problem: A functionally stable internal fixation must be achieved without extensive surgery.

The solution: The hanging fragment is drawn upward by applying the "well-and-bucket" principle. A deltopectoral incision is made, the joint is opened, and the fracture in the cavity floor is reduced. Then a lag screw is driven in through a stab incision made over the spine of the scapula.

Fig. 15a–f. Well-and-bucket effect of a lag screw.
Z.A., ♀, age 19, No. 187928.
a Fracture of the glenoid cavity in a multiple injury patient.
b Downward displacement of the inferior glenoid fragment with fracture in the area of the spina scapulae.
c *Well-and-bucket principle:* The water bucket is hauled upward over a reel.
d *Fracture fixation by this principle:* The lag screw inserted from the crista scapulae into the inferior glenoid fragment pulls the hanging portion upward, thereby reducing the fracture.
e Postoperative roentgenogram.
f *Eight months after injury:* Fracture healed with clinically insignificant incongruity in the glenoid cavity

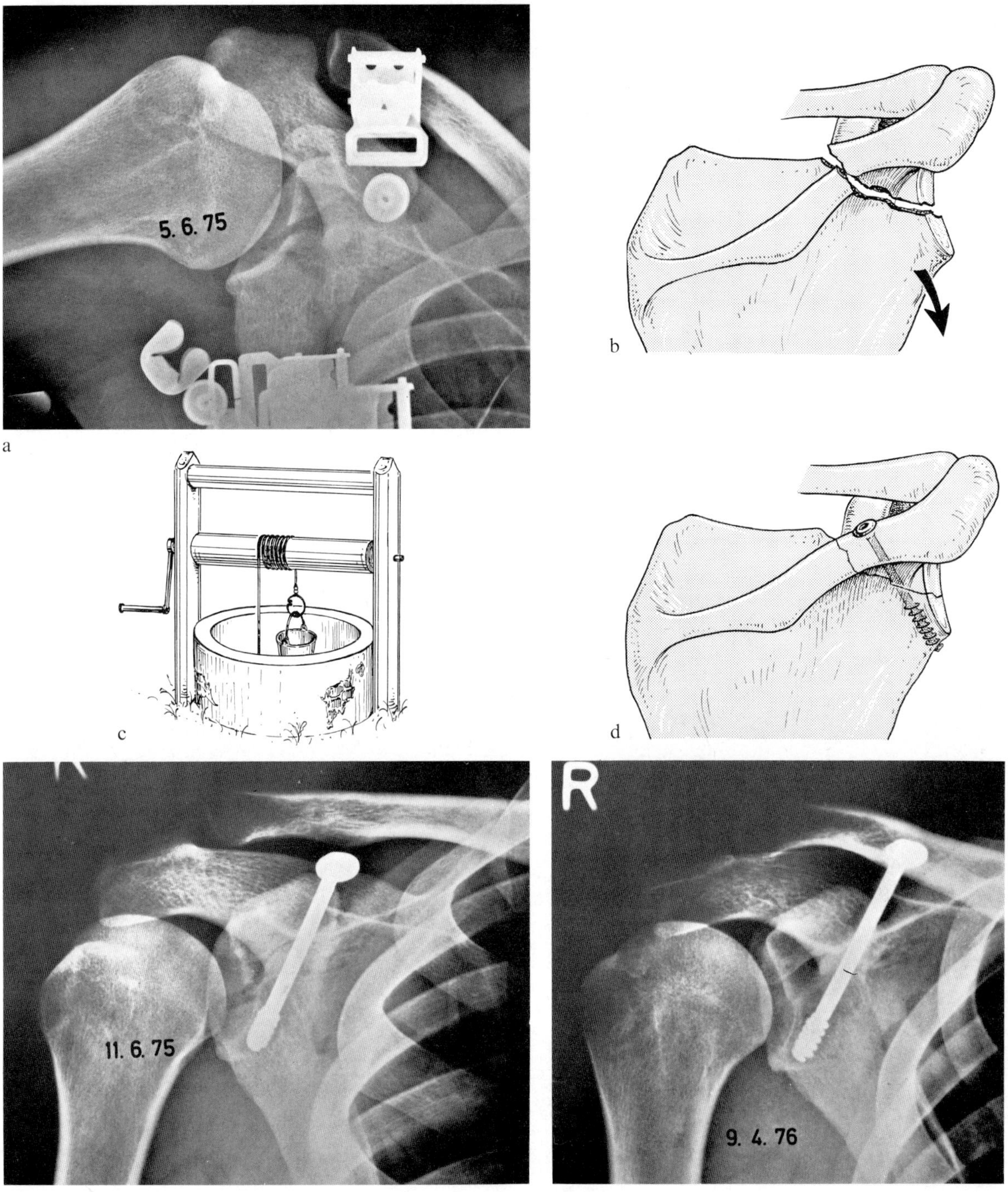
5. 6. 75
a
b
c
d
R
11. 6. 75
e
9. 4. 76
f

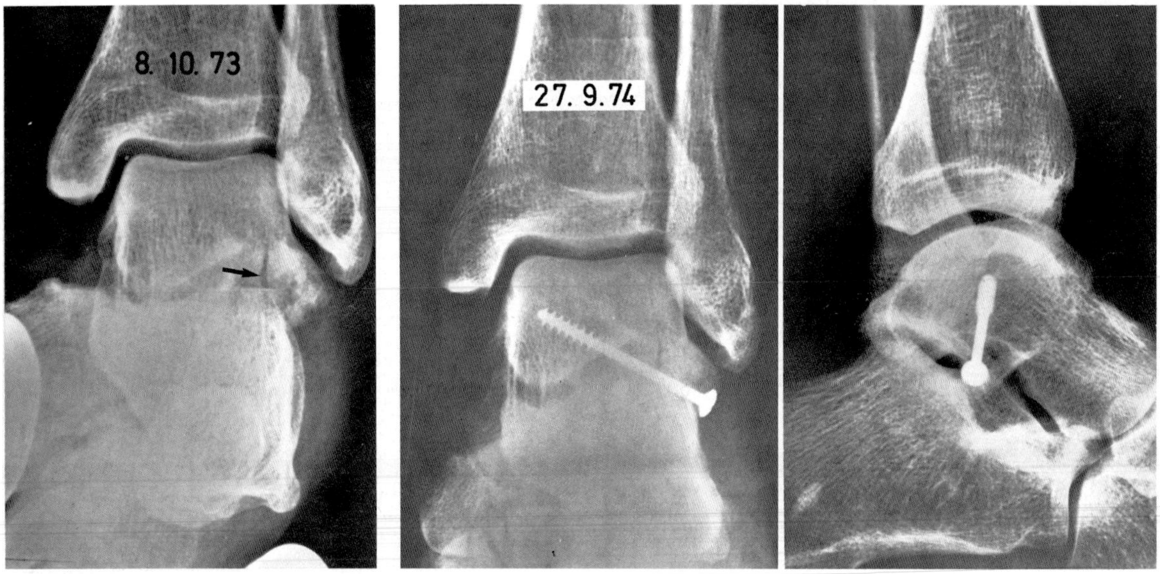

a, b

Example 2: Fracture of the lateral process of the talus (Fig. 16)

The problem: The lateral process bears articular cartilage both superiorly and inferiorly. Its fracture means a loss of congruity in the ankle joint and subtalar joint, which must be corrected.

The solution: From a lateral approach, an arthrotomy is made ventral to the anterior talofibular ligament to assess the quality of the reduction, and is followed by internal fixation with a lag screw.

Fig. 16a, b. Screw fixation of the lateral process of the talus.
K.P., ♂, age 40, No. 171640.
a Avulsion fracture of the lateral process of the talus. Lag screw inserted from the ligament insertion, joint reconstructed.
b *One year after injury:* Complete recovery.

Example 3: Subtalar dislocation (Fig. 17)

Treatment by primary arthrodesis of the subtalar joint is rare, although it will give the best result if there is massive cartilage destruction.

The problem: If cast immobilization is to be avoided, it is necessary to stabilize the freshened joint surfaces by internal fixation.

The solution: From a lateral approach the talocalcanean joints are denuded of cartilage and fixed with screws inserted from below; the calcaneocuboid joint is freed of cartilage and fixed with a Kirschner wire. Aftercare can be administered without external plaster fixation for at least the first 2–3 weeks, until wound healing is complete.

Fig. 17a–d. Screw fixation of the subtalar joint. ▷
H.O., ♂, age 42, No. 173828.
a Subtalar dislocation with massive cartilage destruction.
b *Open reduction of the dislocation:* Affected joints are denuded of cartilage.
c *Postoperative roentgenogram:* Compressive internal fixation of the subtalar joint after cartilage removal, appositional fixation of the calcaneocuboid joint; postoperative mobilization.
d *One year after injury:* Arthrodesis in good functional position

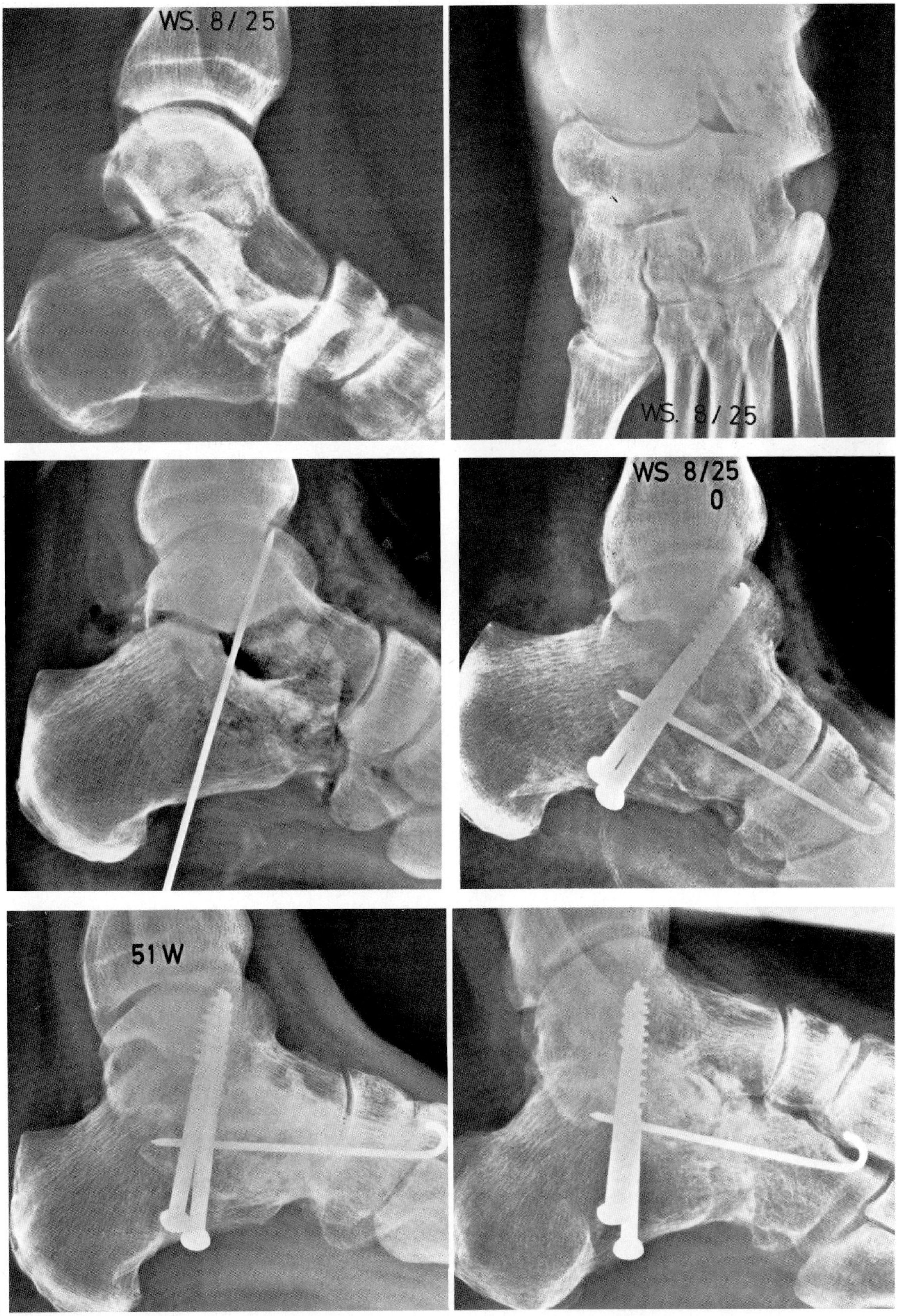

a

b, c

d

1.5 "Hat-hook" Mechanism in Femoral Neck Fractures

Subcapital fractures of the femoral neck are managed in various ways, depending on the situation. In adults with good cancellous bone consistency, open reduction with impaction of the femoral head in valgus anteversion is recommended in order to minimize the risk of pseudarthrosis. The reduction is maintained by screw fixation.

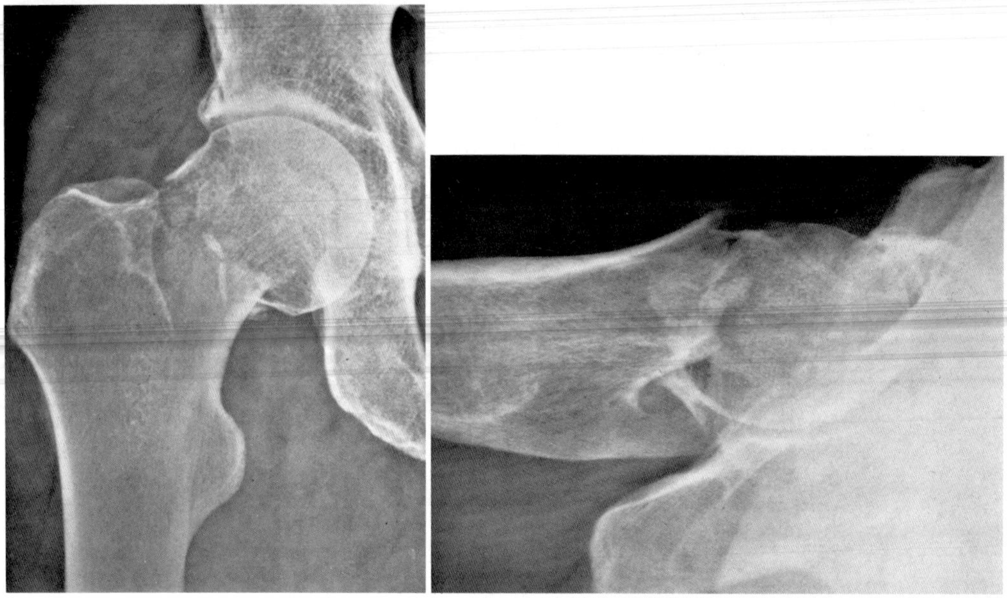

a

Example 1: Subcapital femoral neck fractures in a young patient (Fig. 18)

The problem: The blade of an angled blade plate or a flanged nail would cause microfractures in the very hard cancellous bone of the femoral head, predisposing to necrosis. Anatomic reduction and screw fixation would be unstable because of the comminution of the femoral neck and the shearing forces in the fracture plane.

The solution: After a Watson-Jones incision and arthrotomy, the cancellous bone of the femoral head is curetted to a depth of about 1 cm on the anterocranial side. The head can now be hung onto the spur of the femoral neck like a hat on a hook. Screw fixation compresses the fracture surface, and shearing forces are absorbed by the impacted femoral head.

Fig. 18a–d. Hat-hook reduction of a femoral neck fracture.
I. U., ♂, age 48, No. 190110.
a Subcapital, displaced, and unstable fracture of the femoral neck.
b *Hat-hook principle:* A notch is curetted in the femoral head so that it can be hung onto the hook of the cranial femoral neck spur.
c *Postoperative status:* Femoral head in slight valgus.
d *One year after injury:* Complication-free fracture healing

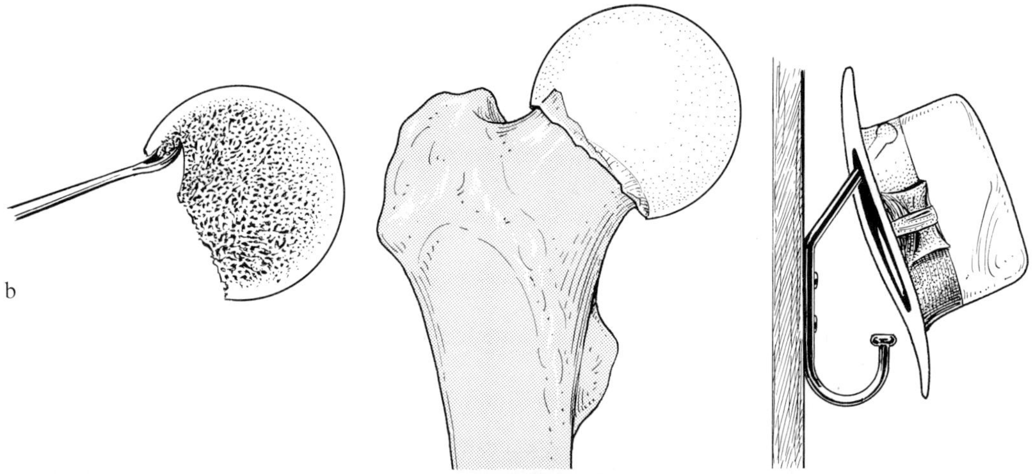

b

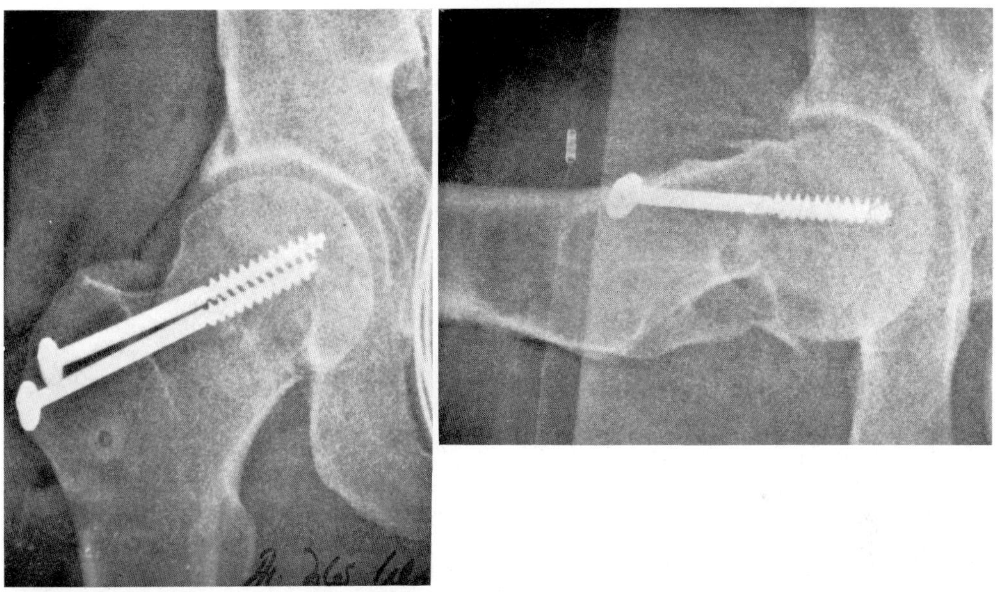

c

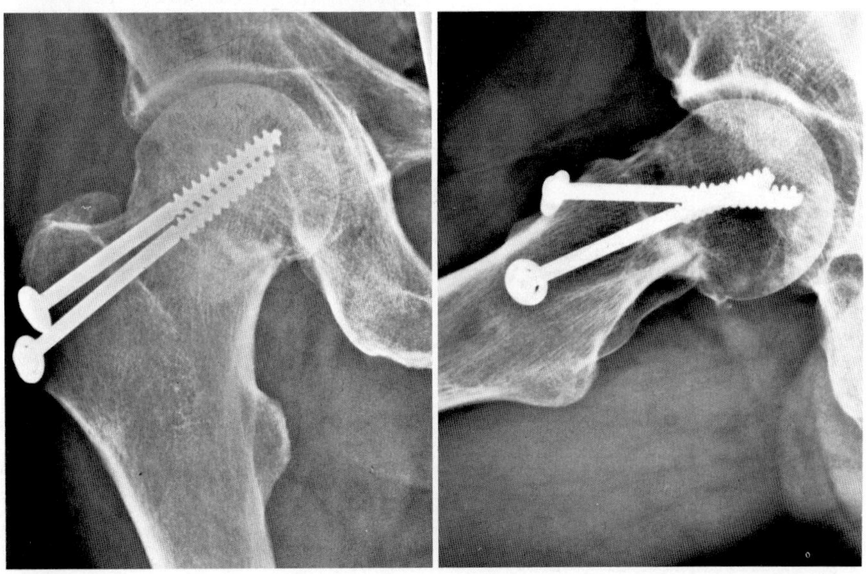

d

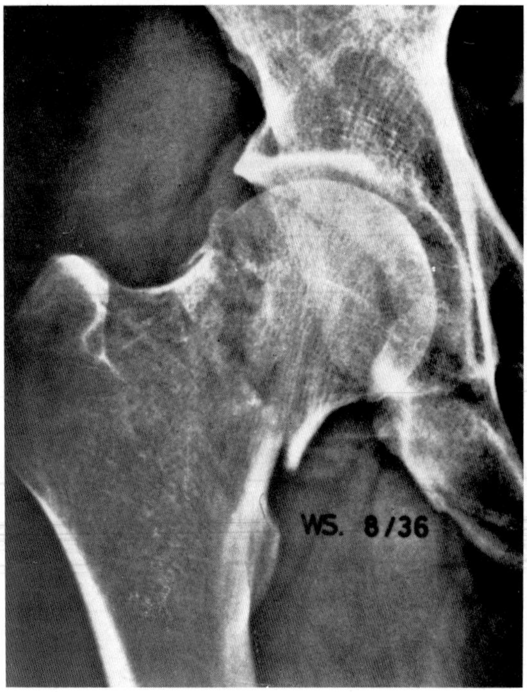

a

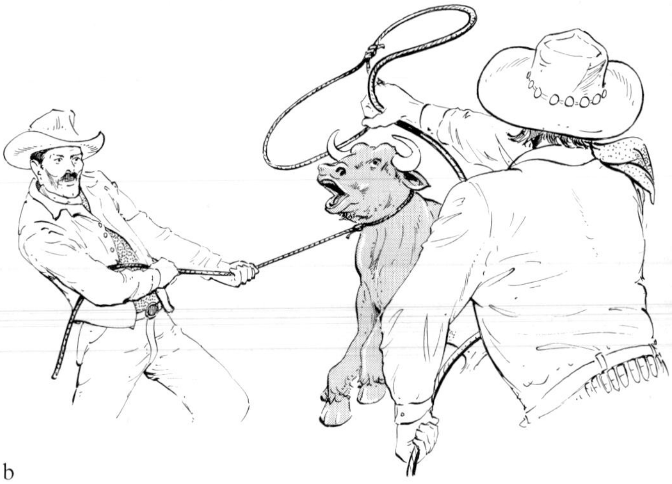

b

Example 2: Subcapital femoral neck fracture with long caudal spur on the head fragment (Pauwels III type fracture) (Fig. 19)

The problem: Due to the vertical course of the fracture plane, shearing forces would remain a problem despite valgus overcorrection and hat-hook impaction of the head. A valgus osteotomy (Pauwels, McElvenny) or the following solution is indicated.

The solution: Following hat-hook impaction of the femoral head, a screw is inserted horizontally downward through the calcar to engage the caudal spur of the femoral neck and keep it from slipping, thus forming a "medial buttress." The lag screws in the upper portion of the head produce stabilizing compression in the fracture plane.

Fig. 19a–e. "Lasso" technique in a femoral neck fracture.
P.G., ♂, age 32, No. 173545.
a Unstable medial femoral neck fracture with long caudal spur.
b *Lasso technique:* First the steer is roped about the neck to prevent his escape, then a second lasso is thrown about his horns to pull him in.
c *Lasso technique + hat hook technique:* The lag screw in the calcar acts like the first lasso to fix the head fragment, then additional lag screws are inserted to "pull it in," i.e., place it in valgus.
d *Postoperative roentgenogram:* Slight valgus overcorrection of the head fragment.
e *Fifteen months after injury:* Uneventful fracture union

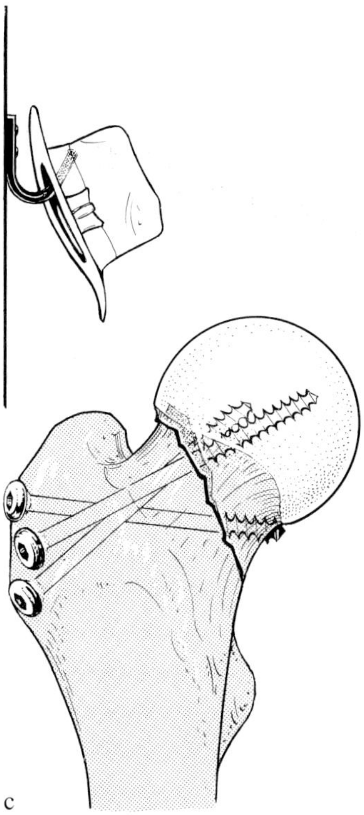

c

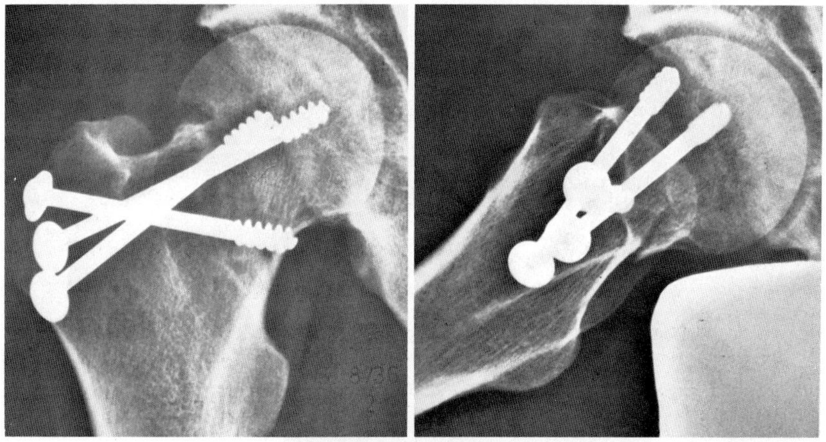

d

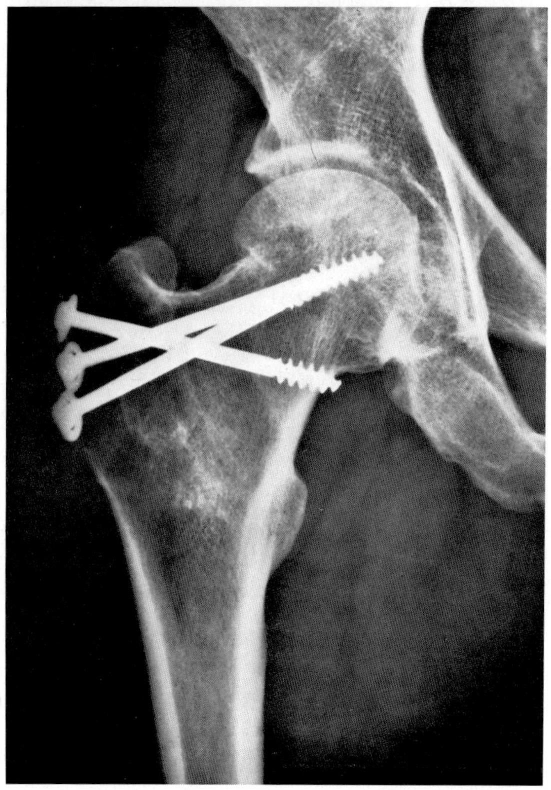

e

2 Wire Loop

2.1 "Tension Band" Wire on the Diaphysis

With tension banding, bending stresses which hamper the reduction of a fracture or osteotomy are converted into pure compressive stresses which act to maintain the reduction. The attendant compressive forces are borne by the fragments, while the tension forces are absorbed by the tension band (plate or wire).

Example 1: Transverse metacarpal fracture with dorsal angulation (Fig. 20)

The problem: The internal fixation should be stable enough to allow postoperative mobilization but should not interfere with the normal function of the extensor tendons. A small tension band plate, dorsally applied, would satisfy the first requirement but would interfere with tendon movements.

The solution: The tension band wire gives excellent fracture stability without compromising tendon function.

Fig. 20 a–d. Tension band loop in a transverse metacarpal fracture.
D.F.V., ♂, age 32, No. 176315.
a *Metacarpal shaft fracture:* Typical angulation due to traction from the palmar muscles.
b *Wire tension band system:* Dorsal traction from the palmar muscles is neutralized by the wire-loop tension band, and the fracture is compressed.
c *Postoperative roentgenogram:* Dorsal figure-of-eight wire loop.
d *Thirteen months after injury:* Complete recovery

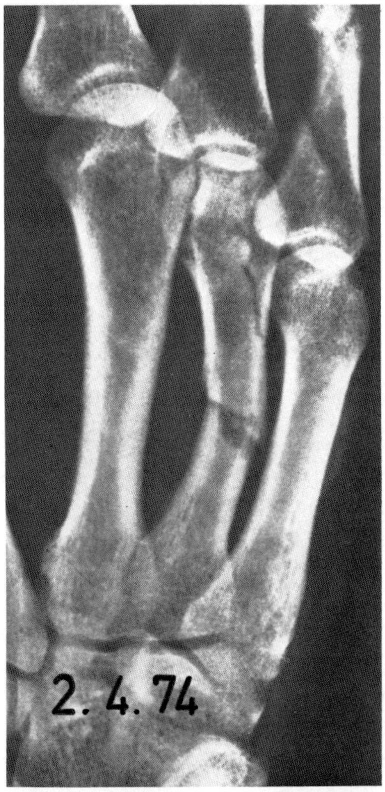

a

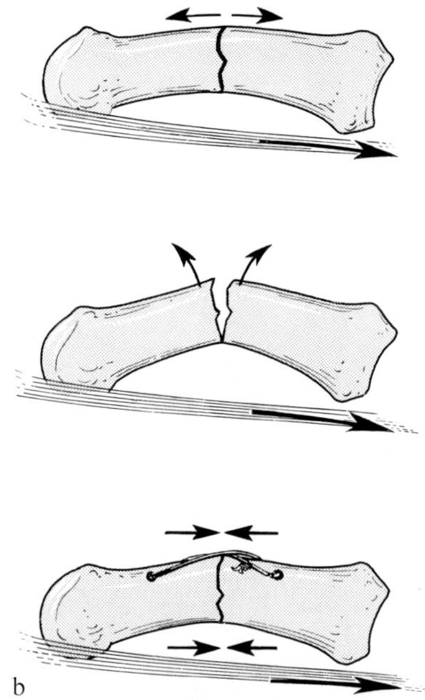

b

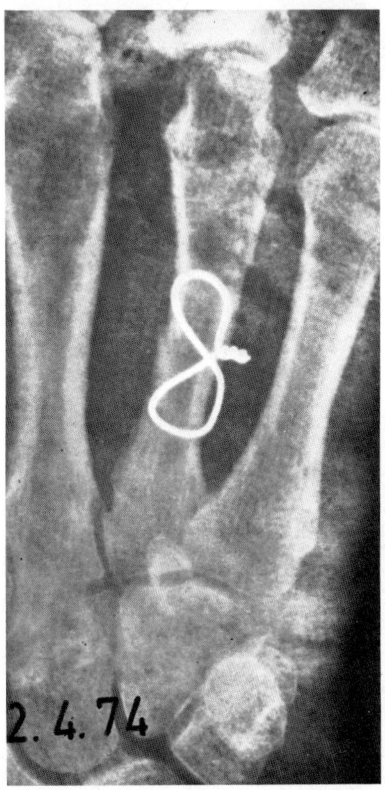

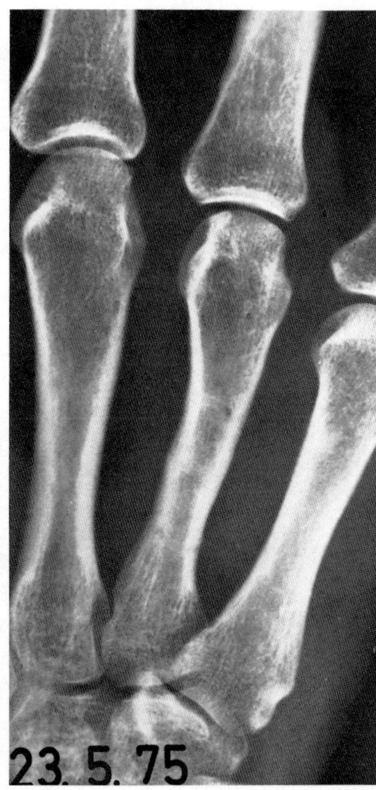

c, d

Example 2: Neglected Monteggia fracture in a child. After treatment of the fracture, correction of the ulna is required (Fig. 21)

The problem: A dorsoradial tension band plate would not only necessitate extensive operative exposure, but also interfere with rotation of the radius.

The solution: The wire tension band adequately stabilizes the wedge osteotomy in the child, especially since a plaster cast can be worn postoperatively without harm. The goal is achieved with minimum effort.

Fig. 21 a–d. Wire tension band in corrective osteotomy of the ulna in a child. H.H.U., ♂, age 7, No. 100361.
a Greenstick fracture of the ulna healed with bowing of the ulna and dislocation of the radial head.
b *Therapy:* Corrective osteotomy of the ulna with radial wedge, internal fixation with wire-loop tension band: radial head spontaneously reduced.
c *Four months after osteotomy:* Ulna healed, radial head in correct relation to capitulum of humerus.
d *Seven years after osteotomy:* Complete recovery

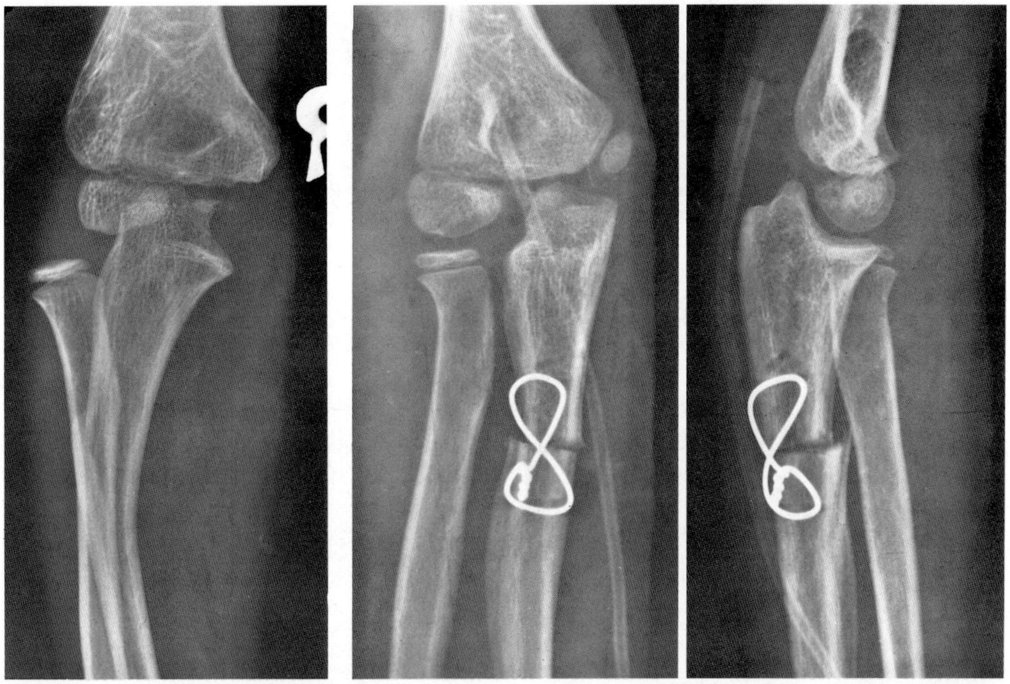

a, b

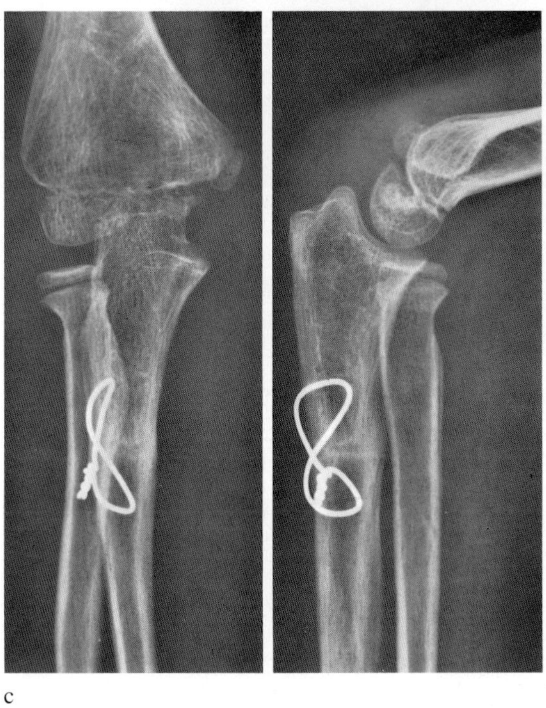

c

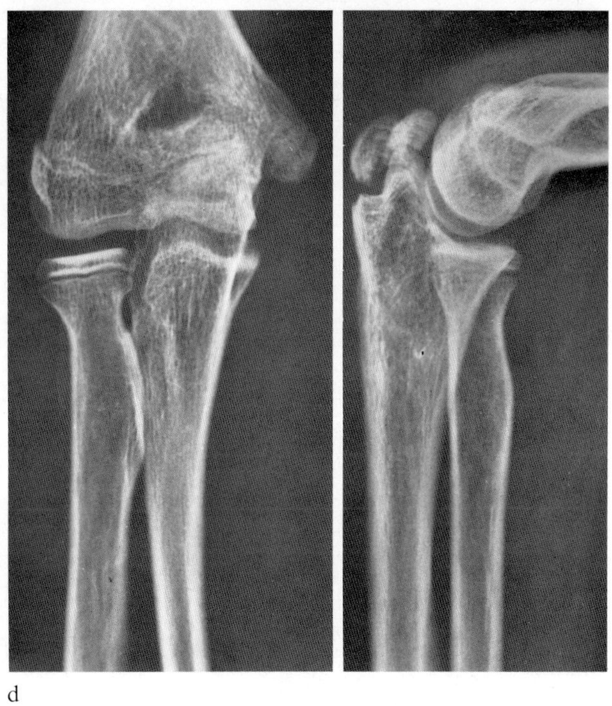

d

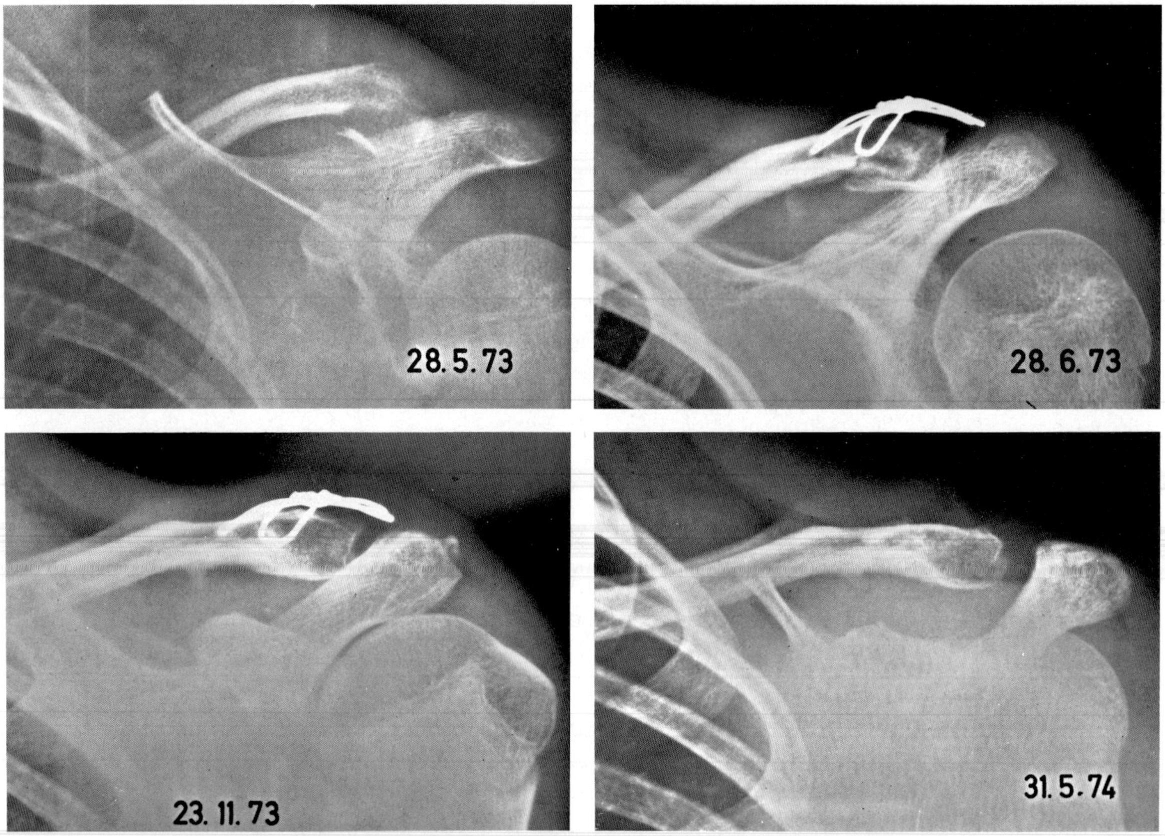

a, b

c, d

Example 3: Extreme lateral clavicular fracture with small distal fragment (Fig. 22)

The problem: Fixation cannot be achieved with plates or Kirschner wires.

The solution: A double wire tension band anchored in two channels drilled through the central fragment indirectly engages the peripheral fragment. The wires engage the joint capsule in the same way in which the triceps tendon is engaged in fractures of the olecranon.

Fig. 22a–d. Tension band wiring of a lateral comminuted fracture of the clavicle.
T.R., ♂, age 17, No. 168296.
a Lateral comminuted fracture of the clavicle.
b *Operation:* Open reduction, double tension band wiring. The wires are anchored in the joint capsule peripherally and in drilled channels centrally.
c *Six months after injury:* Fracture healed without complications.
d *One year after injury, after removal of implants:* Complete recovery

a–c

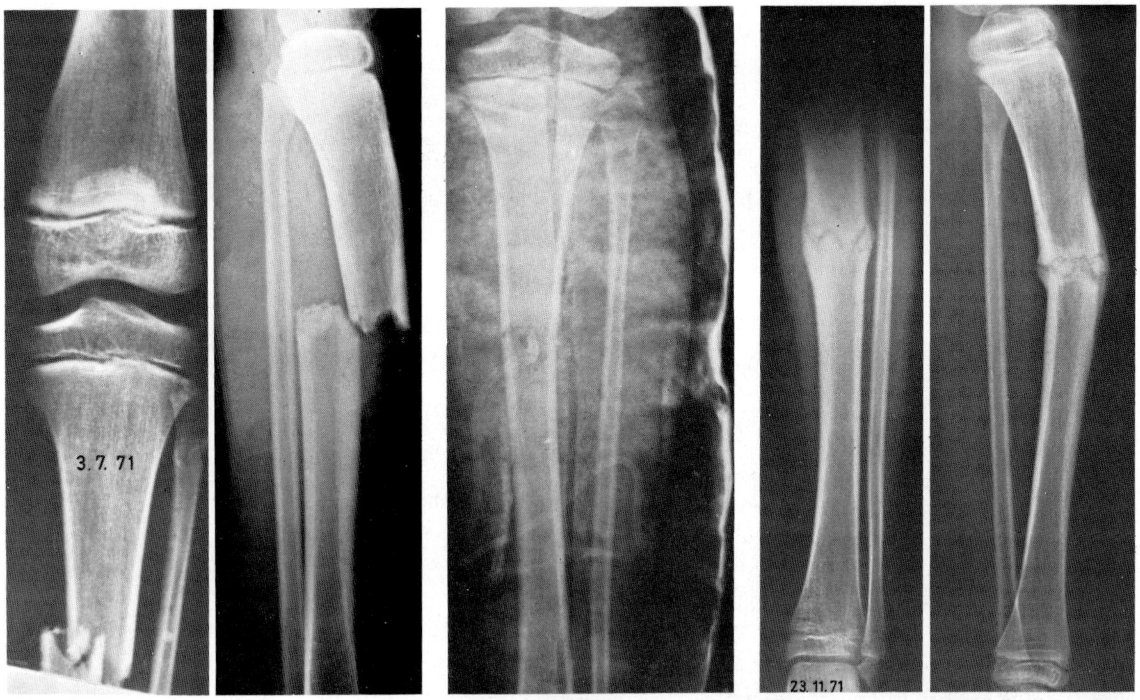

d, e

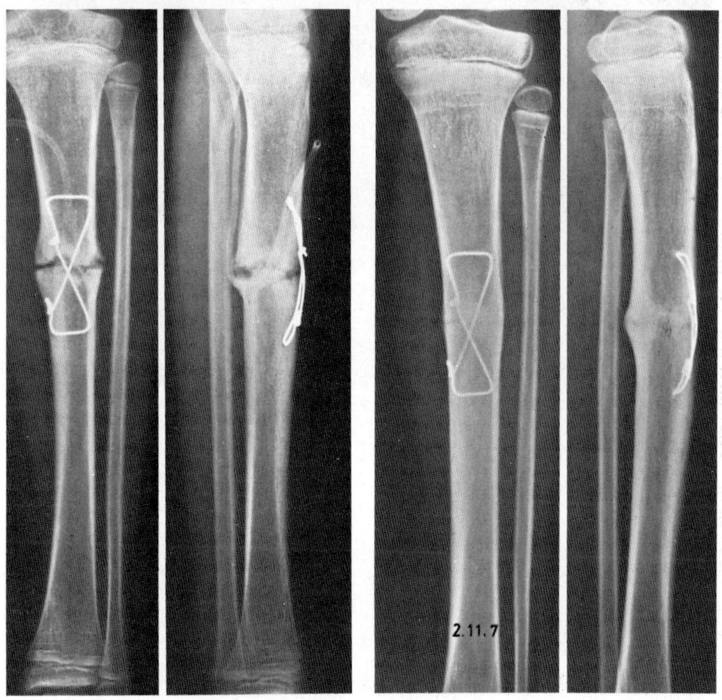

Fig. 23a–e. Tension band wiring of tibial pseudarthrosis with anterior angulation in a child.
S.J., ♀, age 7, No. 150698.
a Second-degree open tibial fracture.
b *Therapy:* Conservative treatment in plaster cast.
c *Four months after injury:* Hypertrophic tibial pseudarthrosis with anterior angulation.
d *Operation:* Mannual correction of angular deformity, simple figure-of-eight wire loop used as tension band.
e *One year after operation:* Pseudarthrosis healed without deformity

Example 4: Hypertrophic pseudarthrosis of the tibia with anterior angulation in a child (Fig. 23)

The problem: In the rare cases of tibial pseudarthrosis in children, as little foreign material as possible should be implanted in order to avoid undesired growth stimulation.

The solution: The wire tension band offers an ideal solution to this problem.

2.2 Tension Band Wire on the Vertebral Column

With kyphotic instability, a posterior tension band wire offers the simplest means of correcting an unstable deformity.

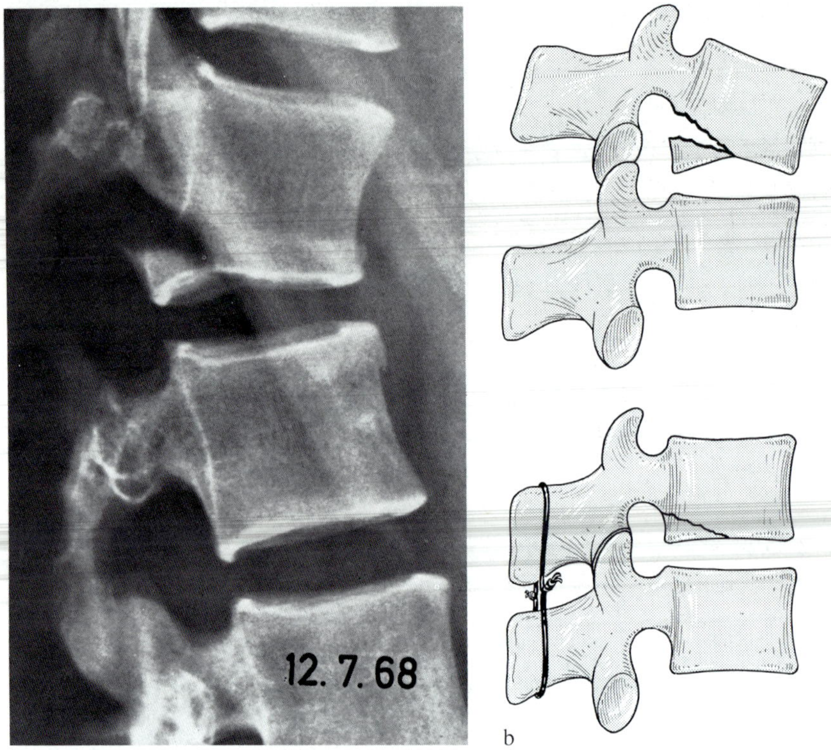

a b

Example 1: Fracture-dislocation with subluxation of the facets and loosening of the intervertebral disc (Fig. 24)

The problem: The ruptured posterior elements (ligaments, muscles) have to be replaced to permit postoperative mobilization of the spine.

The solution: The spinous processes are bound together with a wire loop from a posterior approach.

Fig. 24a–d. Tension banding of an unstable fracture-dislocation of L-1 with subluxation of the facets.
G.G., ♀, age 21, No. 127248.
a Fracture-dislocation of L-1 with massive subluxation of the L-1–L-2 facets.
b *Operative technique:* The facet subluxation is reduced by hyperextension of the spine, and an interspinous tension band stabilizes the reduced fracture.
c *Postoperative status.*
d *Seventeen months after injury, one year after wire removal:* Only low-grade disc narrowing, osseous recovery complete

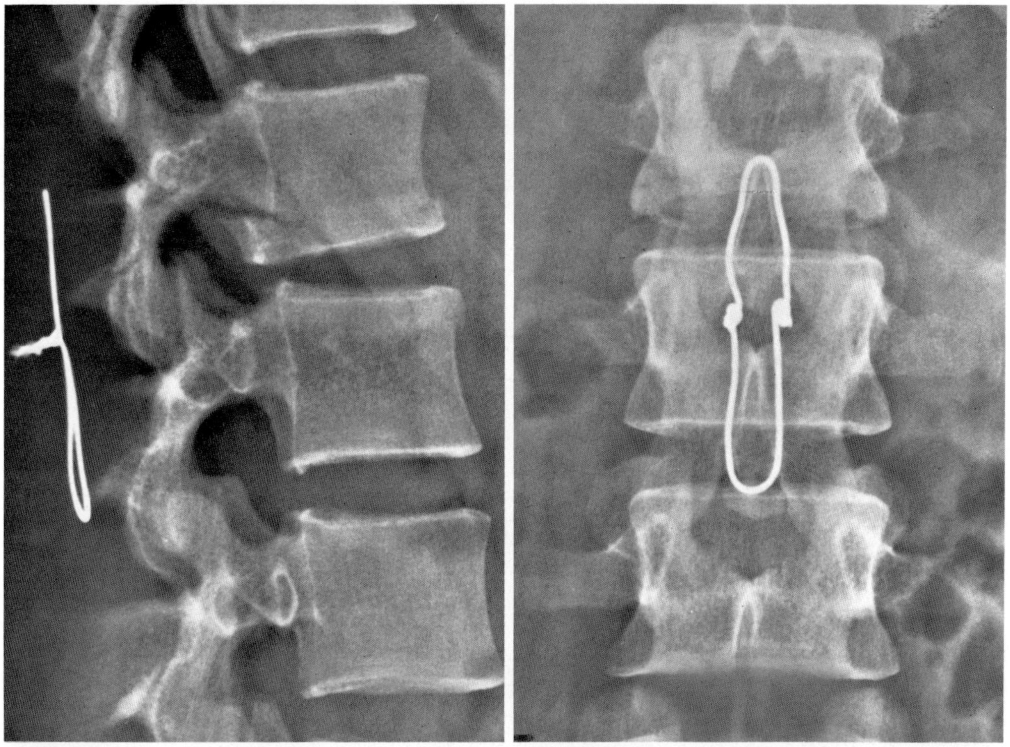

c

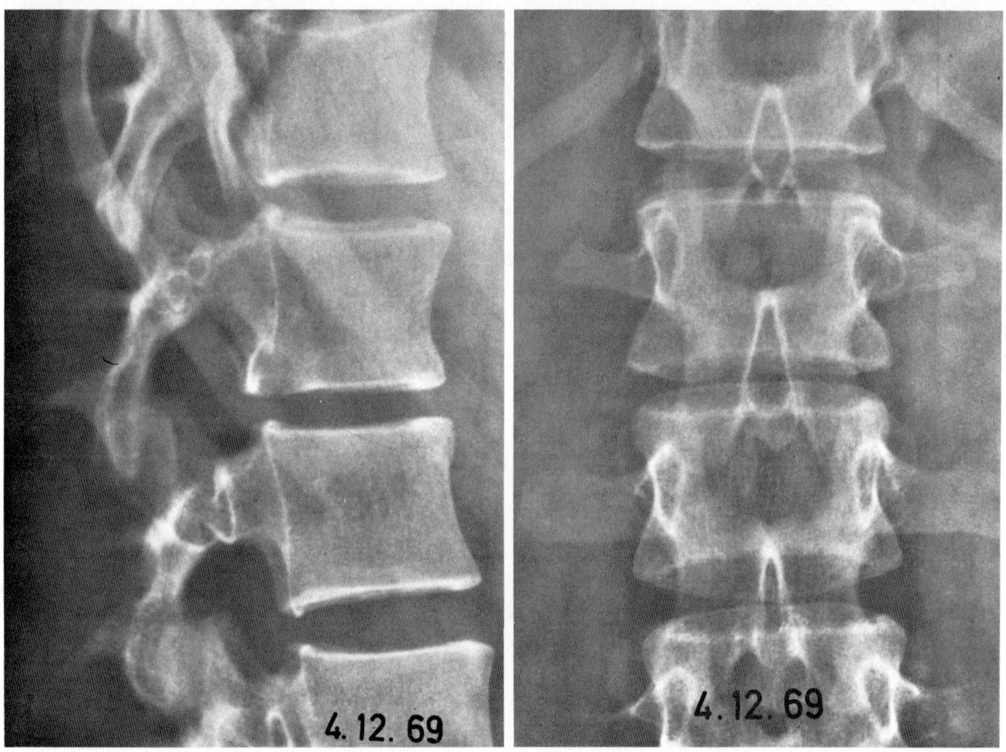

d

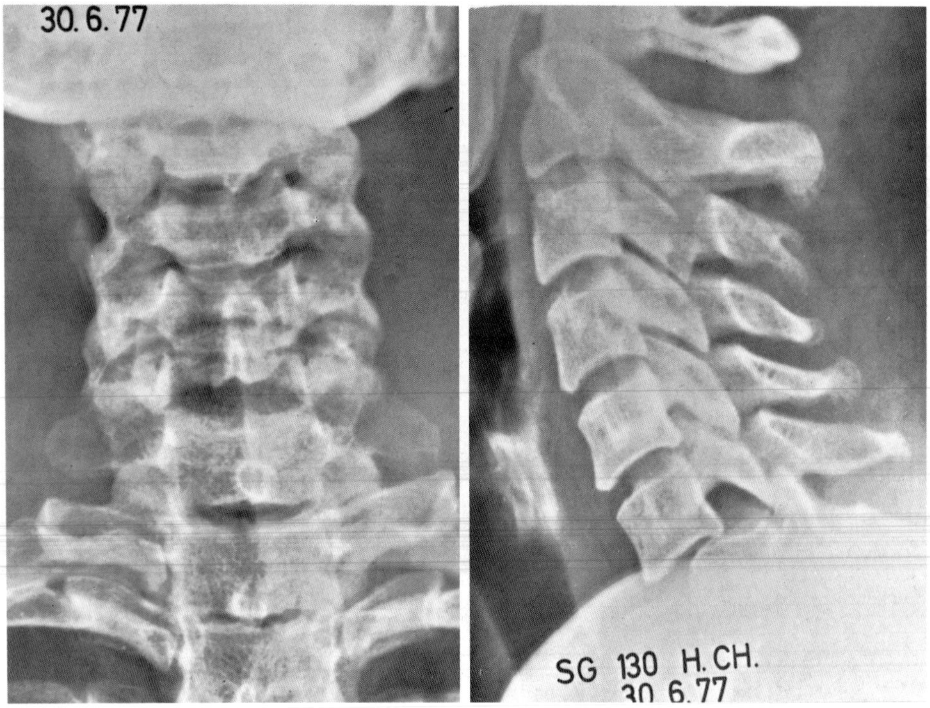

a

Example 2: Dislocation of the cervical facets with ligament rupture (Fig. 25)

The problem: Because the posterior ligamentous elements are ruptured, there is a danger of kyphotic deformity after reduction. The posterior ligament function must be replaced until fibrous strengthening occurs.

The solution: Open reduction from a posterior approach, followed by tension band wiring of the spinous processes.

Fig. 25a–c. Temporary wire fusion in a dislocation of the cervical spine.
H.C., ♀, age 30, No. 209372.
a Dislocation of C-6–C-7 with facet locking and paraparesis.
b *Operation:* Open reduction of the locked facets, suturation of the ligaments. The reduction is stabilized with a wire tension band anchored cranially around the C-6 lamina and caudally around the C-7 spinous process.
c *One year after injury:* Marked disc narrowing resulting from trauma-related disc lesion, facet joints stable. The partially ruptured wire may be removed.

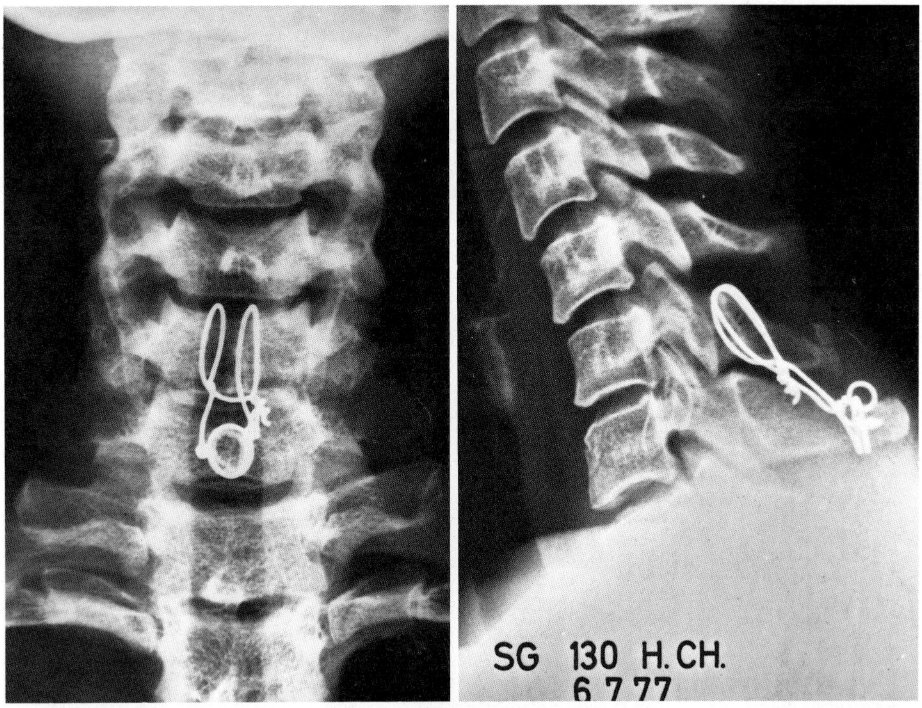

b

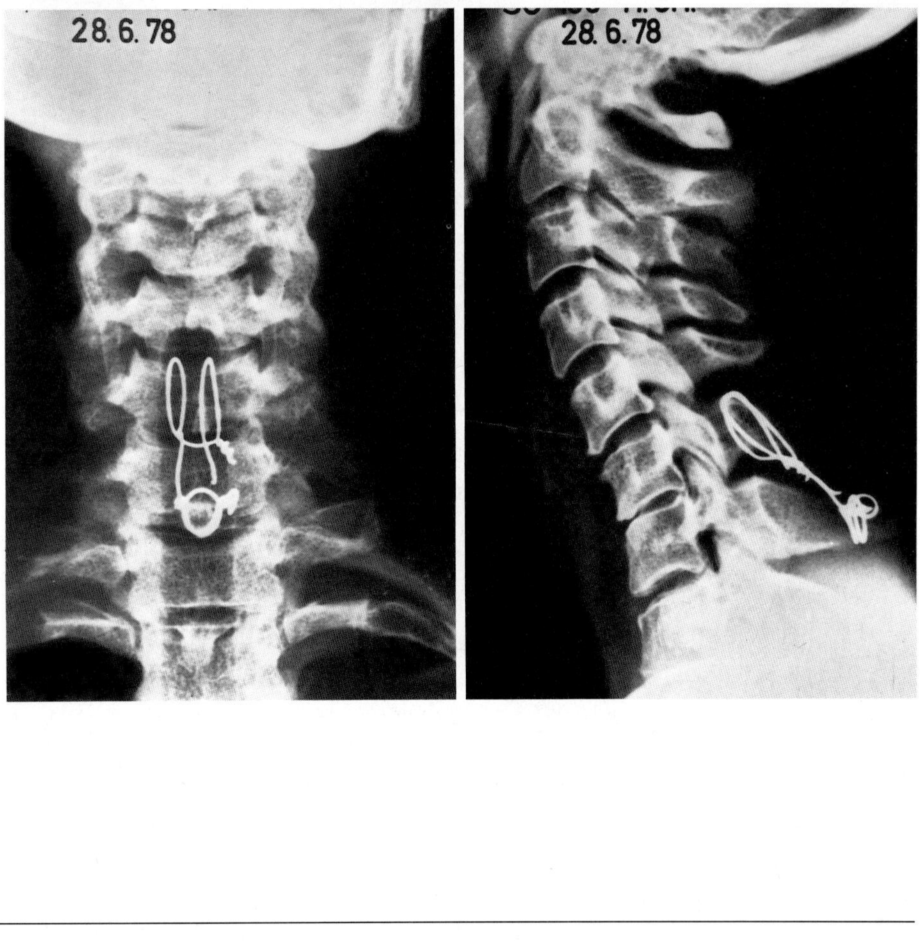

c

2.3 Wire Loop in Ligament or Tendon Insertion

The wire loop is the implant of choice for the internal fixation of certain avulsion fractures.

Example 1: Traumatic rupture of the symphysis pubis with marked separation (Fig. 26)

The problem: Rigid closure of the separation is mandatory due to the attendant sacroiliac dislocation. Rigid plates almost always loosen, because the elastic pelvic girdle requires a dynamic symphyseal suture.

The solution: The wire loop in the tendon insertions of the gracilis muscles provides a sufficiently dynamic hold to stabilize the rupture. Under the protection of the wire loop, the ligament injuries in the area of the symphysis and sacroiliac joint can heal undisturbed.

Fig. 26a–d. Stabilization of a traumatic symphyseal rupture with a wire loop. B.H., ♂, age 49, No. 155663.
a Separation of the symphysis with dislocation of the sacroiliac joints.
b *Principle of operation:* The pubic bones can be reapproximated by the "shutter latch" mechanism.
c *Operation:* The wire loop in the tendon insertions of the two gracilis muscles fixes the symphyseal rupture and permits healing of the soft tissue lesions.
d *Four months after injury:* The symphysis and sacroiliac joints are again stable

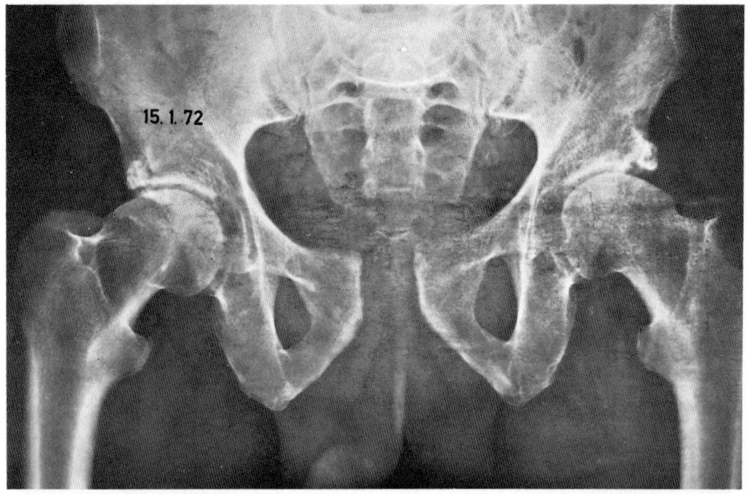

a

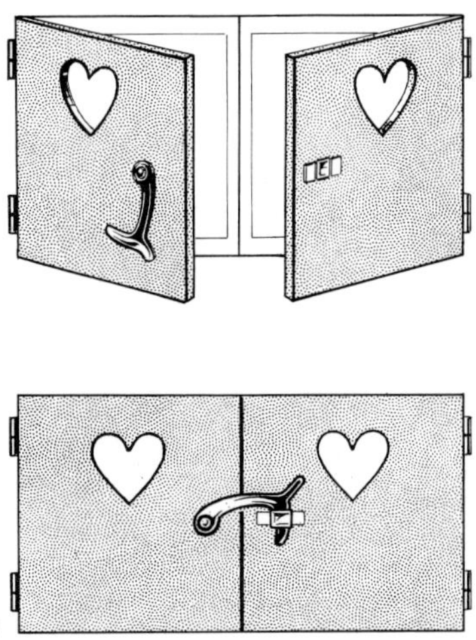

b

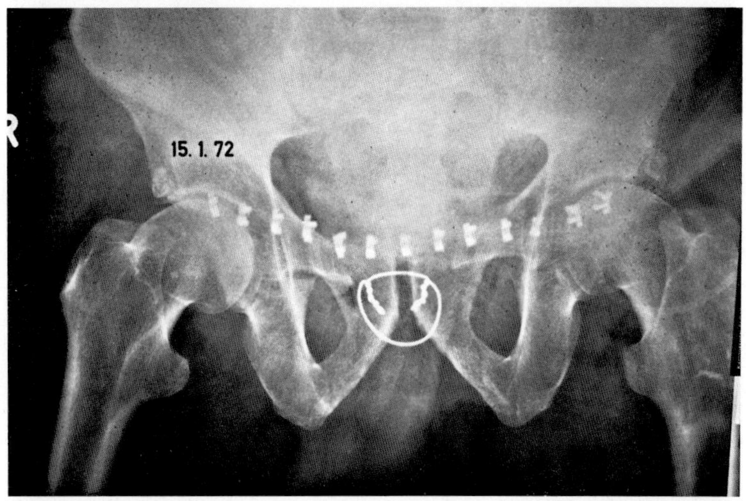

c

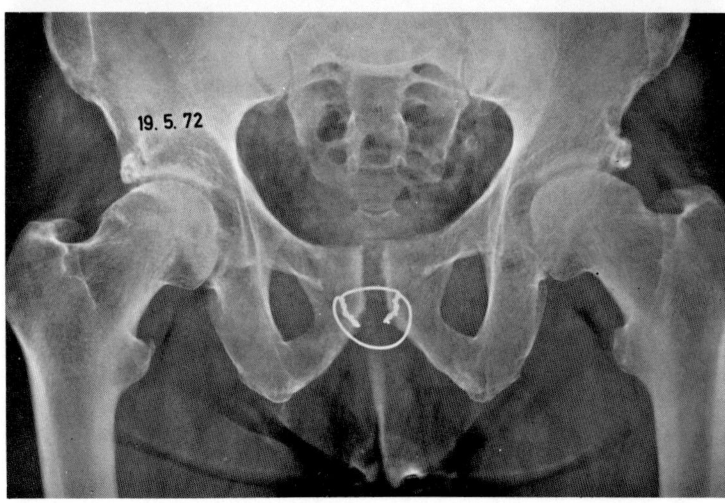

d

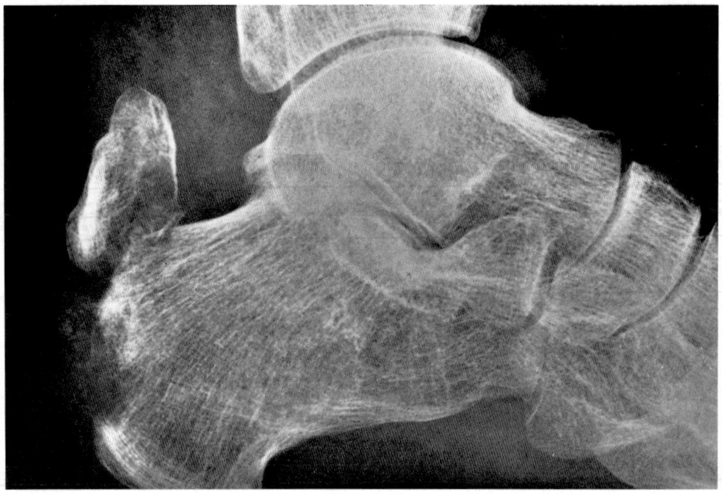

a

Example 2: Achilles tendon avulsion fracture (Fig. 27)

The problem: The small fragment cannot be stabilized with a screw. Moreover, only small incisions may be made to gain access to the fracture.

The solution: Through a lateral para-achilles incision, the fragment is reduced, and a wire loop is applied over it. With the aid of a curved cannula and three small stab incisions, the wire is crossed in figure-of-eight fashion and pulled through beneath the calcaneus, so that it is firmly anchored in the origin of the plantar aponeurosis. This technique allows postoperative mobilization.

Fig. 27a–d. Fixation of an Achilles tendon avulsion fracture with a wire loop. N.F., ♂, age 36, No. 141557.
a Displacement of bony tendon insertion.
b *Operative technique:* After a para-achilles skin incision, the wire is made to encircle the calcaneus and tendon insertion in figure-of-eight fashion with the aid of a cannula and several stab incisions. Tension forces are stably neutralized.
c *Postoperative roentgenogram.*
d *Five months after injury:* Complete recovery

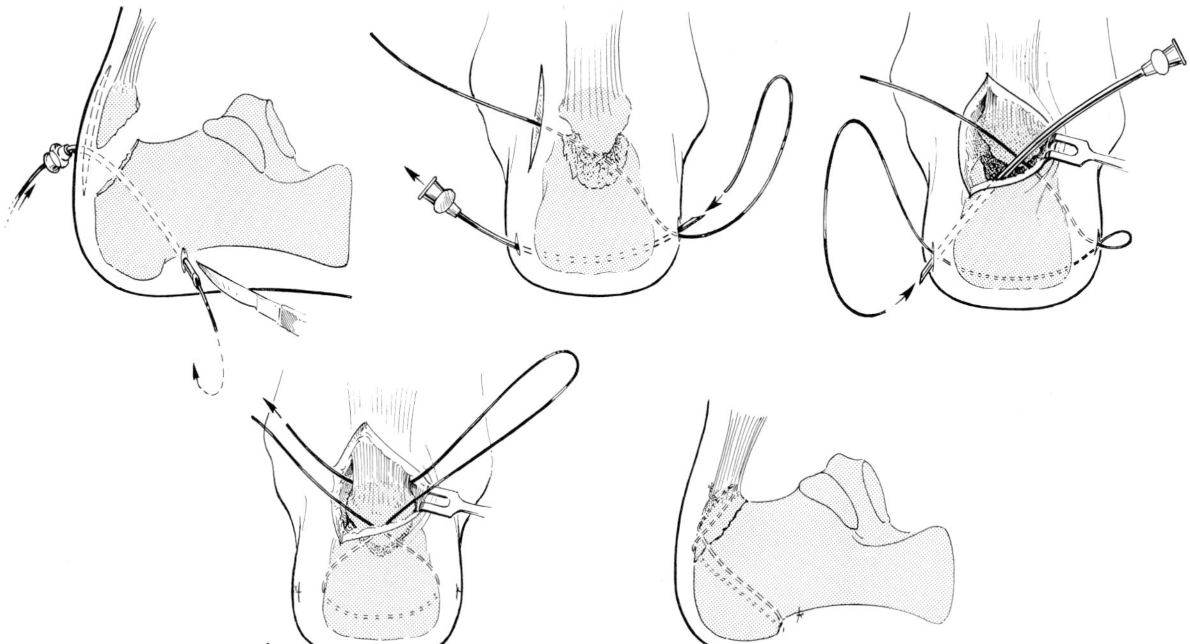

b

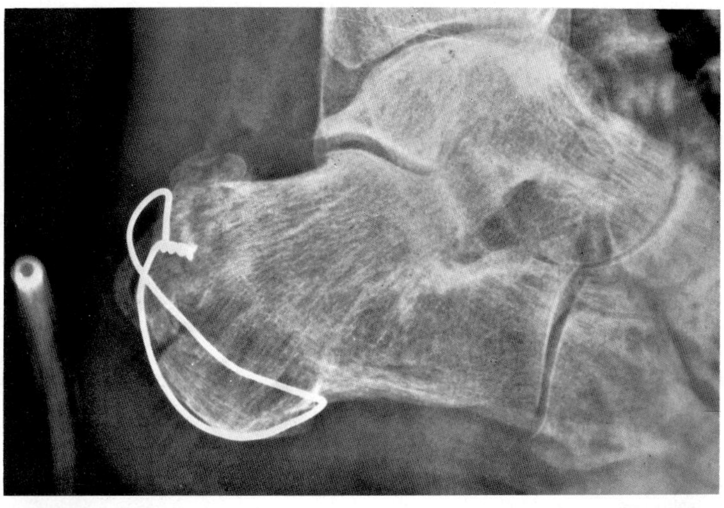

c

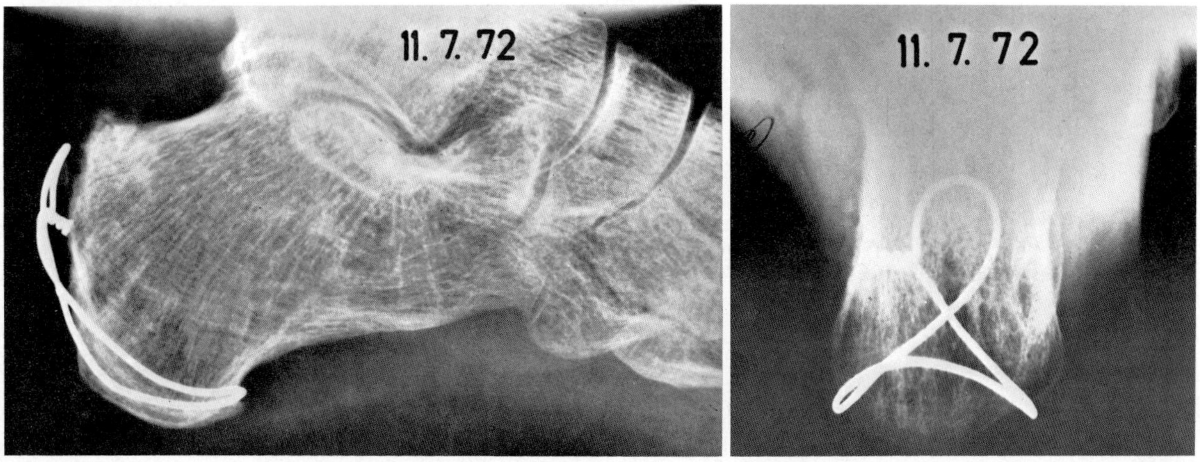

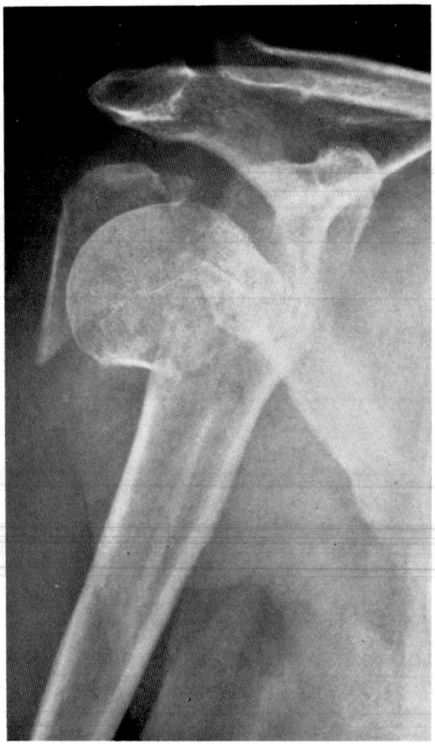

a

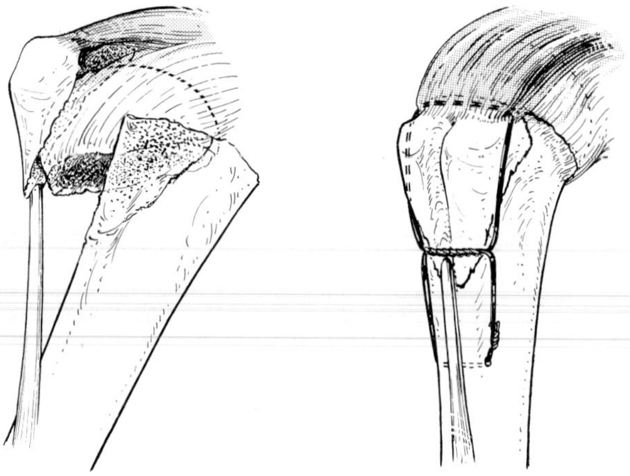

b

Example 3: Subcapital fracture of the humerus with avulsion of both tubercles (Fig. 28)

The problem: We know of no conventional internal fixation technique (screws, plates) for managing this type of comminuted fracture.

The solution: From a deltopectoral approach the wire loop is passed through the tendon insertions of the rotator cuff on both tubercles. The shaft of the humerus is approximated to the head, and the rotator cuff is drawn against the shaft with the wire loop. This fixation allows postoperative mobilization, and the fracture unites without secondary varus angulation.

Fig. 28a–d. Wire-loop tension band in a subcapital humeral fracture with avulsion of both tubercles.
E.H., ♀, age 59, No. 154287.
a Fracture-dislocation with avulsion of the tubercles.
b *Scheme of operation:* The shaft is impacted into the head fragment, the tubercles are reduced against the shaft, and a wire-loop tension band is applied which engages the rotator cuff.
c *Postoperative status.*
d *Four months after injury:* Fracture is healed

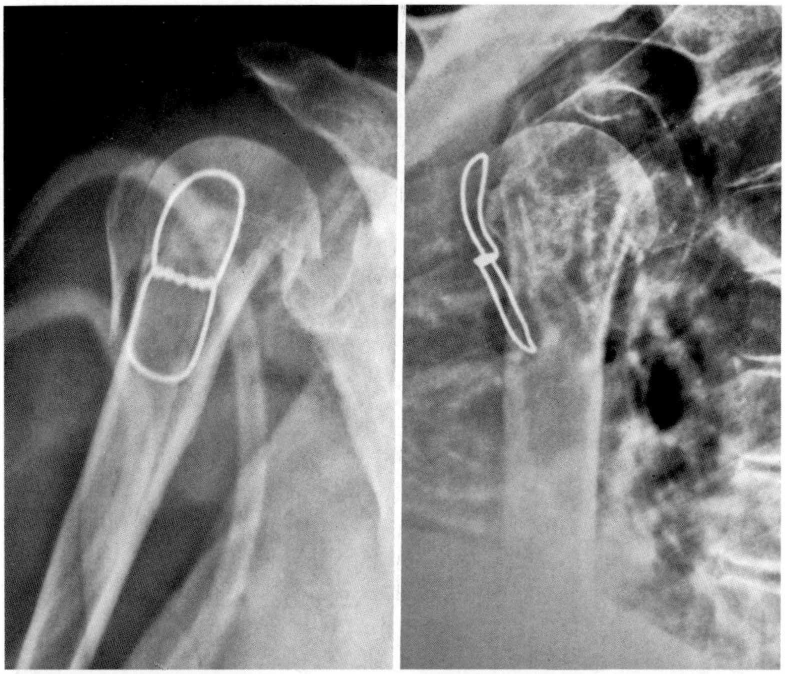

c

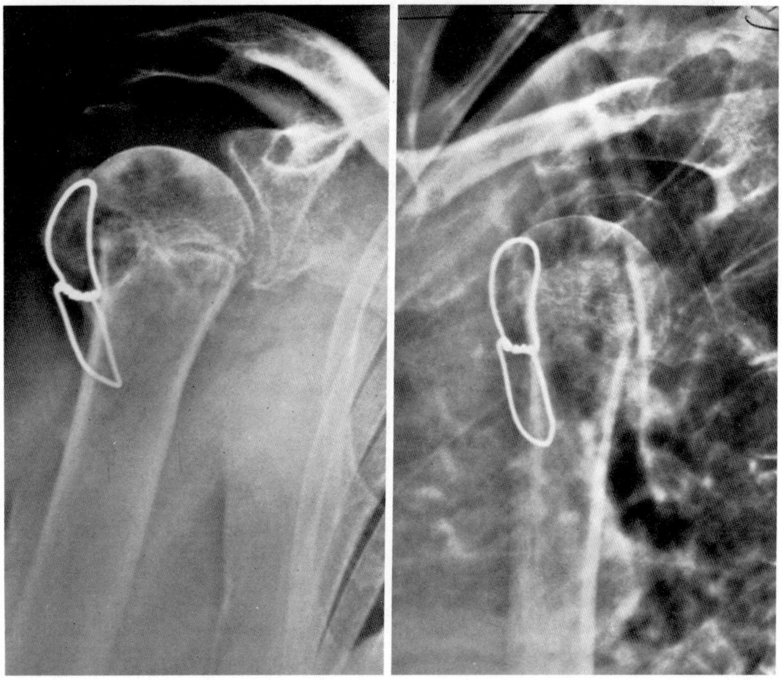

d

Example 4: Flaccid pseudarthrosis following humeral osteotomy (Fig. 29)

The problem: A faulty osteotomy performed for recurrent dislocation of the shoulder has resulted in pseudarthrosis with dislocation of the humeral head. The rotator cuff is lax, and the bone is porotic.

The solution: After removal of the old implants, the humeral head is reduced on the shaft in valgus. Each tubercle is engaged with a wire loop passed through the tendon insertions of the rotators. The wires are passed distally around a screw with washer and tied off securely. The rotators are again under tension, which serves to maintain reduction of the humeral head. Under the protection of the tension band, the pseudarthrosis heals without further immobilization and without bone grafting.

Fig. 29a–c. Tension band wiring of a subcapital humeral pseudarthrosis. G.F., ♀, age 56, No. 196522.
a Condition after rotation osteotomy for recurrent shoulder dislocation: pseudarthrosis, severe osteoporosis, dislocation of the shoulder joint.
b *Tension banding:* After removal of the old implants, two wire loops are passed through the rotator cuff insertions on the tubercles, then brought distally around the head of a cortex screw with washer to form a tension band. An additional fragment is fixed by cerclage.
c *Eleven months after operation:* Pseudarthrosis is healed, shoulder function is satisfactory

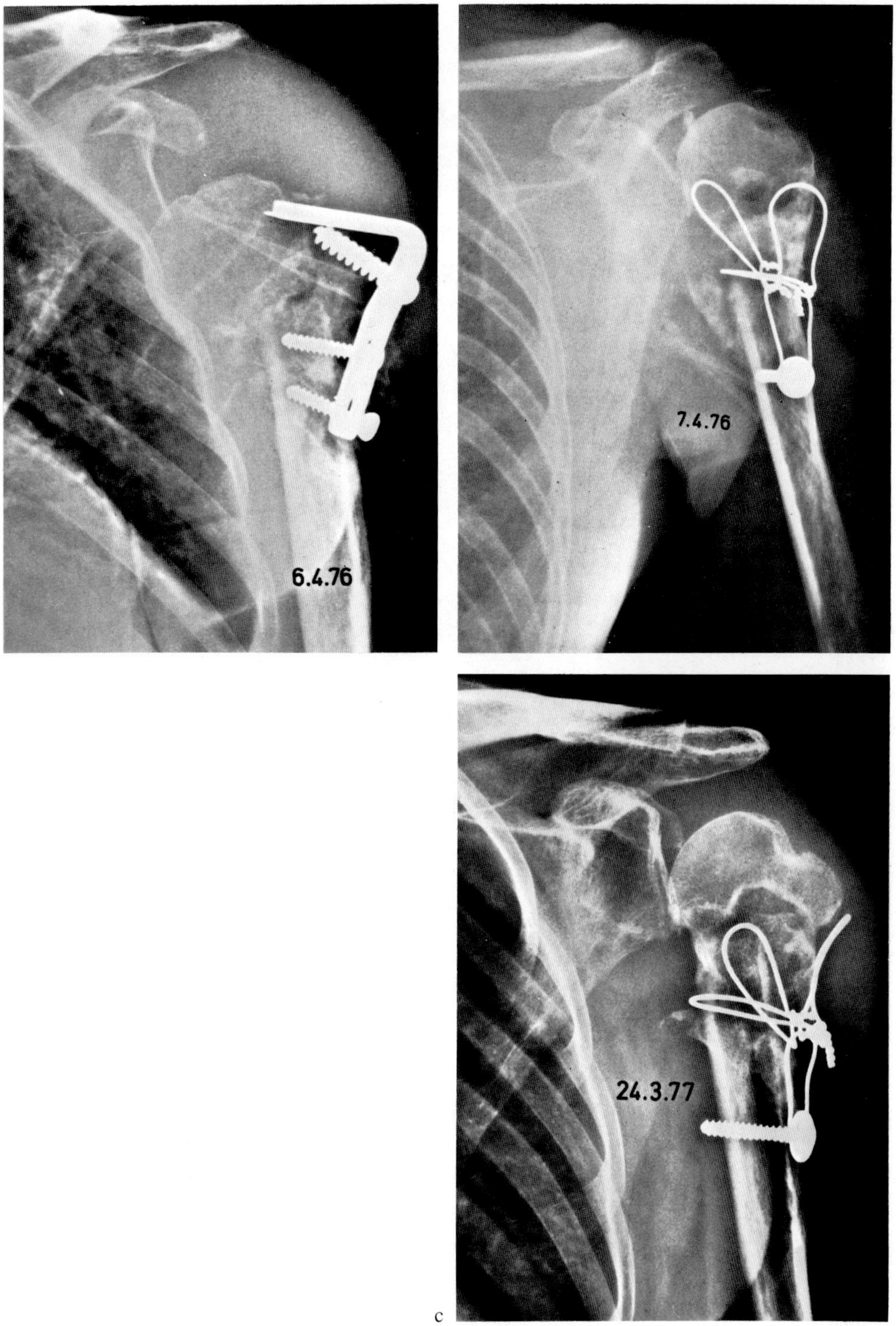

a, b

c

Example 5: Avulsion fracture of the tuberosity of the fifth metatarsal bone (Fig. 30)

The problem: The internal fixation should allow postoperative mobilization and must therefore counteract the pull of the peroneus brevis tendon.

The solution: The fracture is anatomically reduced by means of a small wire loop passed through the tendon insertion proximally and through a drill hole in the fifth metatarsal distally. The wire tension band ensures undisturbed fracture healing.

Fig. 30a–c. Tension banding of an avulsion fracture of the tuberosity of the fifth metatarsal bone.
C.D., ♀, age 31, No. 121974.
a *Intra-articular fracture:* The fragment is displaced by traction from the peroneus tendon.
b Wire loop is passed proximally through the tendon insertion and distally through a drill hole in the shaft.
c *Twenty-two weeks after injury:* Fracture is anatomically healed, recovery is complete

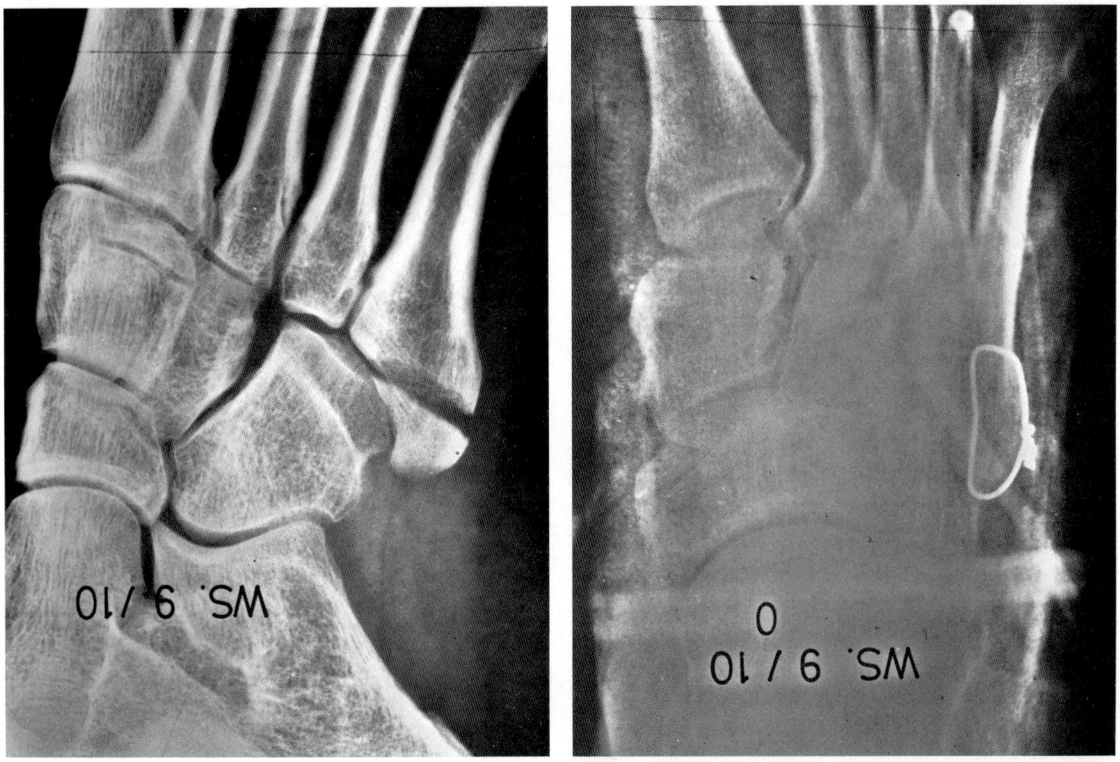

a, b

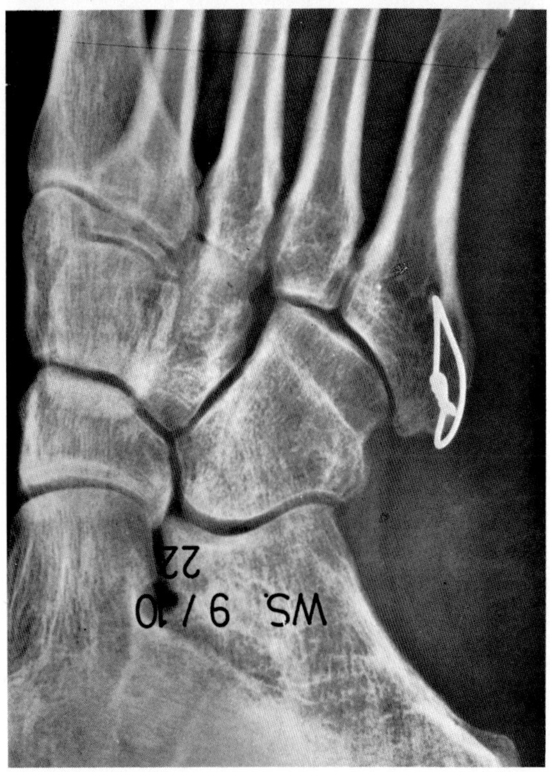

c

2.4 Wire Loop to Secure a Tendon or Ligament Suture

Tendon or ligament sutures should be protected against overstretching for the first 6–8 weeks. In cases where immobilization is undesirable or impossible, there is a danger that the suture will tear or the ligament will elongate with a loss of function. A wire loop capable of bearing dynamic loads can protect the suture in such cases until the substrate is sufficiently revascularized to withstand the tensile forces.

Example 1: Dislocation of the sternoclavicular joint (Fig. 31)

The problem: Dislocation of the sternoclavicular joint is more than just a cosmetic problem, especially in manual laborers and athletes. Suture of the torn short ligaments and rigid joint capsule is not sufficient to maintain the reduction. Only by temporarily tethering the clavicle to the first rib can adequate stability be obtained. Additional stabilization is necessary so that the sutured ligament and tether (strip of fascia lata) can heal without disturbance.

The solution: The ligament suture and fascia lata tether are protected by a wire loop, which is also passed around the clavicle and the first rib. The wire loop is removed after 3 months.

Fig. 31 a–c. Syndesmoplasty protected with wire loop in sternoclavicular dislocation.
S. I. G., ♀, age 20, No 184524.
a Functionally and cosmetically troublesome medial dislocation of the clavicle.
b *Operation:* Open reduction and dynamic stabilization of the clavicle by a fascia lata strip anchored to the first rib. Syndesmoplasty is secured with a wire loop around the clavicle and first rib.
c *Six months after injury:* Perfect functional and cosmetic result

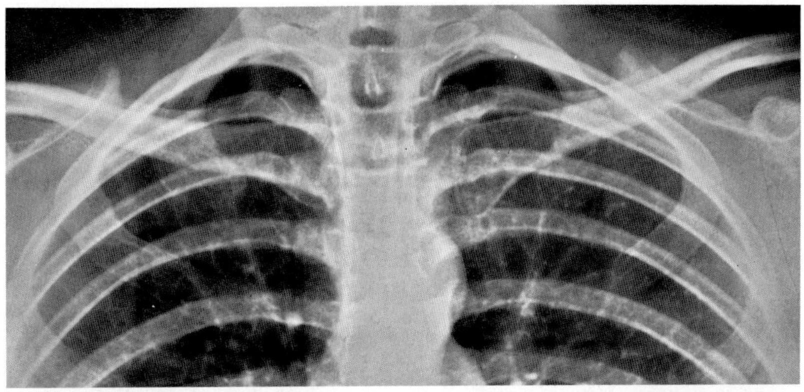

a

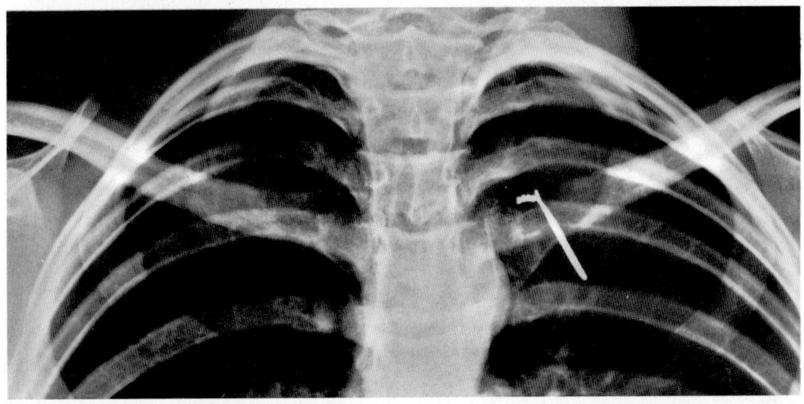

b

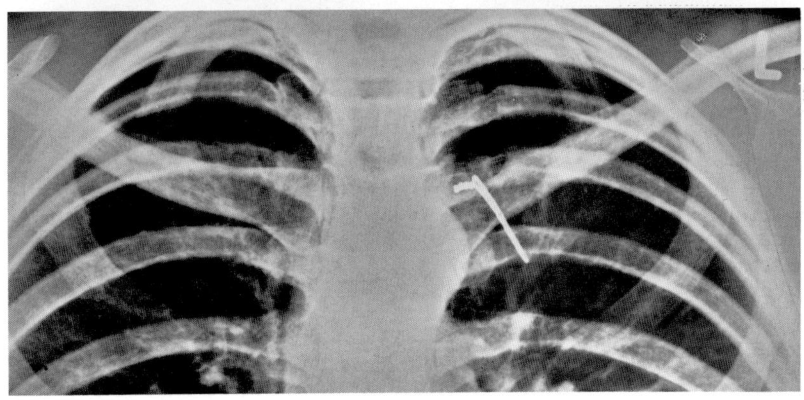

c

a

b

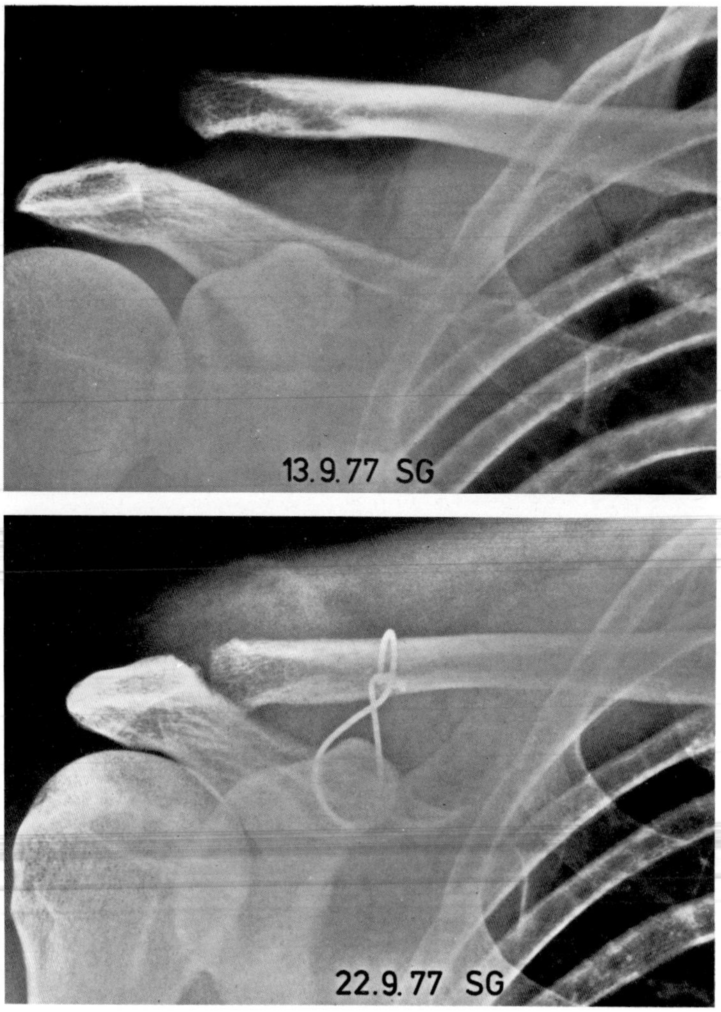

Fig. 32a, b. Ligament replacement protected by wire loop in acromoclavicular dislocation.
H.K., ♂, age 47, No. 209317.
a Old acromioclavicular dislocation.
b *Operation:* Coracoclavicular ligament replacement with m. plantaris tendon, protected by wire loop around the clavicle and coracoid process

Example 2: Recurrent dislocation of the acromioclavicular joint: coracoclavicular ligament replacement (Fig. 32)

The problem: The transplant between the clavicle and coracoid process should remain unstressed for 8–10 weeks to promote its revascularization.

The solution: The transplant, which consists of a plantaris tendon or fascia lata strip sutured to itself, is dynamically protected by the wire loop until revascularization is complete. The wire will succumb to fatigue fracture at 8–10 weeks, but by then the transplant should be fully functional.

2.5 Wire Loop as Cortical Bone Suture

In selected cases a simple wire loop can provide a simple solution for, or contribute to the solution of, an internal fixation problem.

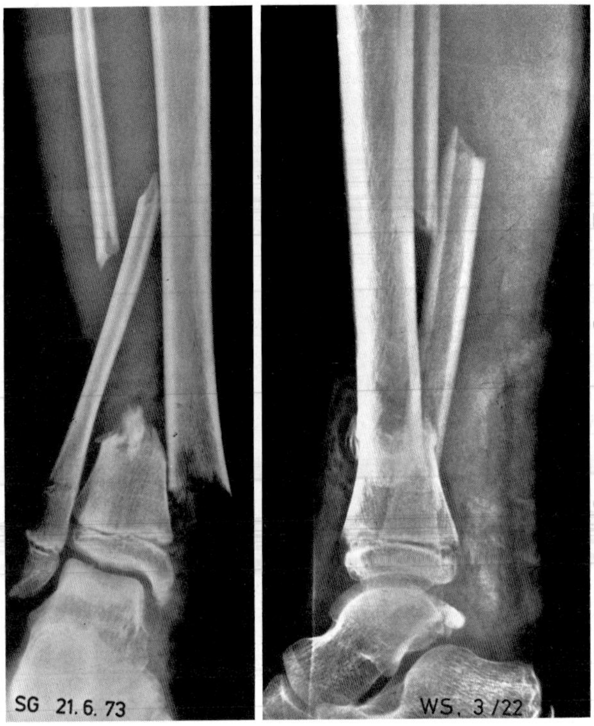

a

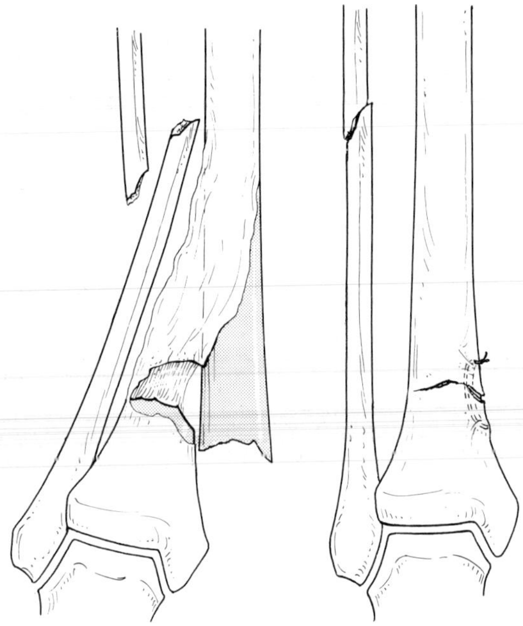

b

Example 1: Open fracture in a child with intact periosteum on one side (Fig. 33)

The problem: The massive soft tissue destruction on the medial side of the tibia prohibits internal fixation with bulky implants (plate).

The solution: Following reduction, a small wire loop is applied transosteally. Stability is provided by the combined support of this loop and of the intact lateral periosteum.

Fig. 33a–e. Cortex wire suture. H. M., ♀, age 9, No. 168939.
a Second-degree open fracture.
b *Internal fixation technique:* The reduced fracture is stable as soon as the medial periosteum is replaced. This is done with the wire suture.
c *The wire loop functions as a padlock:* Once the lock is in place, the box cannot be opened.
d *Postoperative roentgenogram:* Anatomic reduction.
e *One year after injury:* Fracture healed without complications

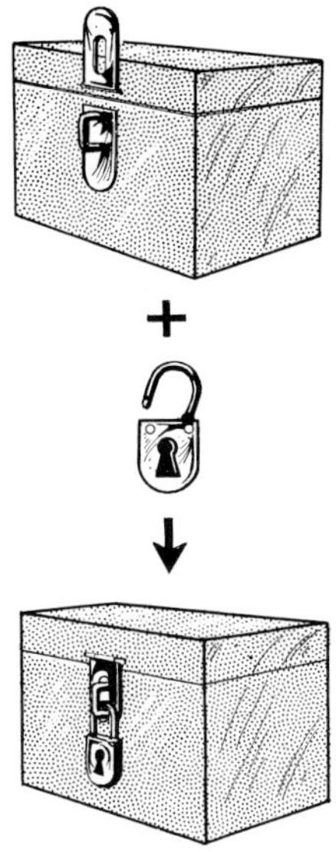

c

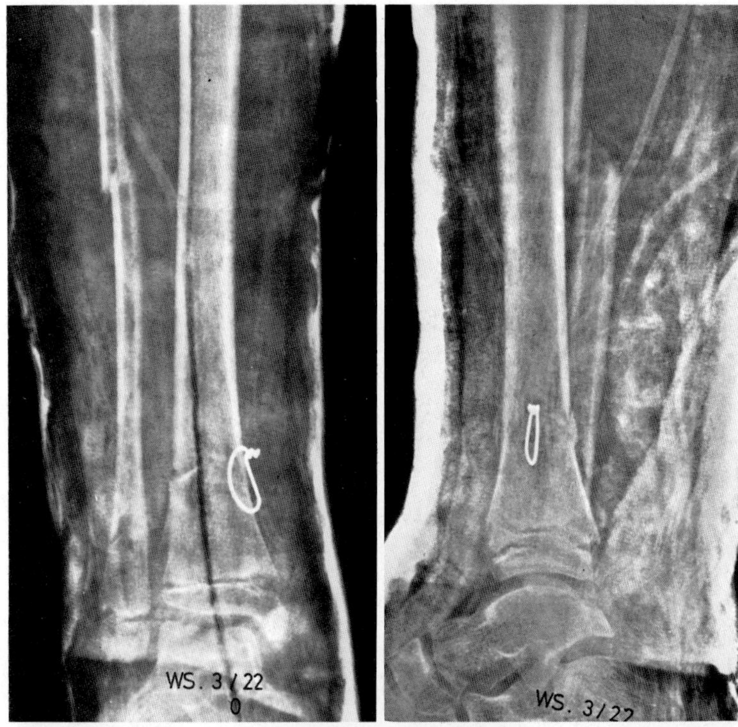

d

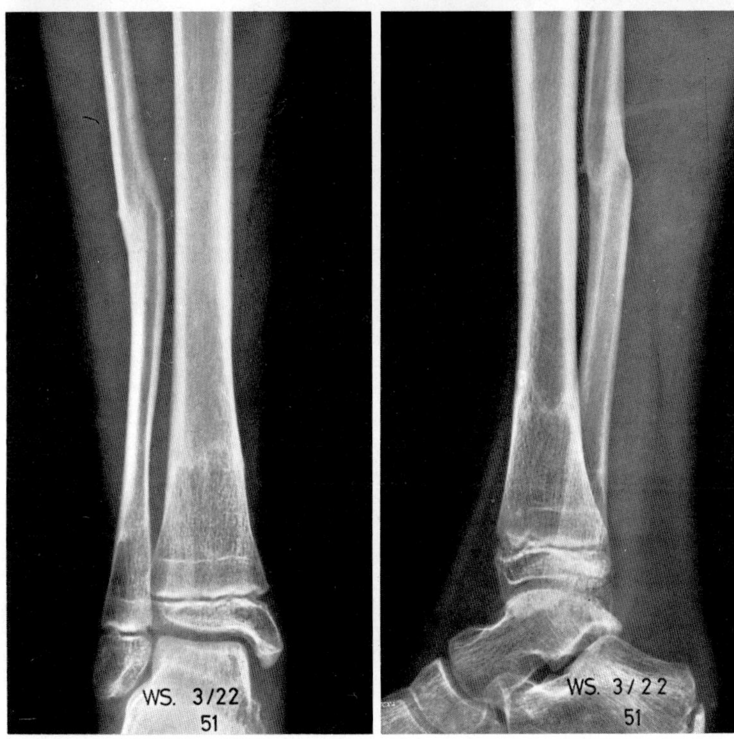

e

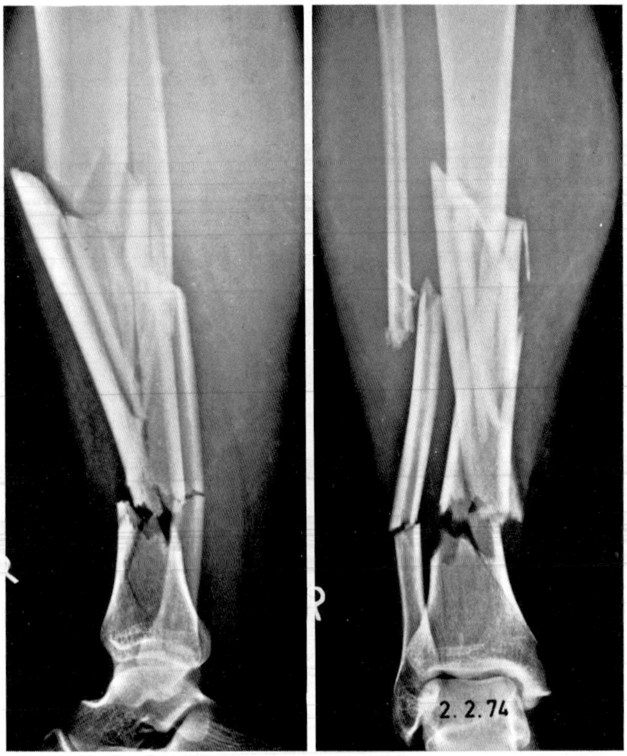

a

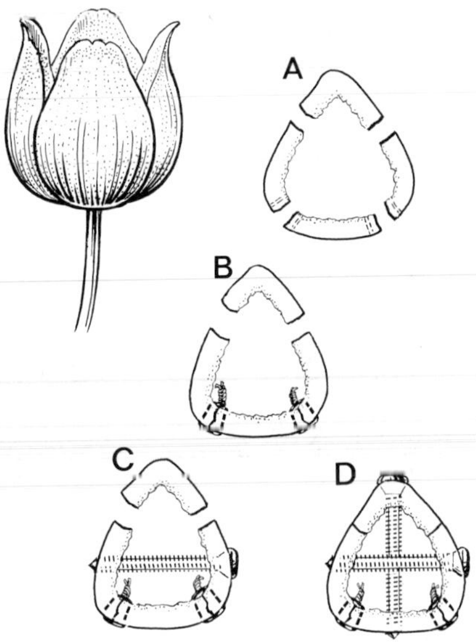

b

Example 2: Segmental comminuted fracture of the lower leg with incipient anterior tibial compartment syndrome (Fig. 34)

The problem: This is an emergency situation requiring broad operative splitting of the fascia of the compartment. Thus, a stable internal fixation becomes all the more important for optimum aftercare of this serious soft tissue injury. However, the all-important intermediate fragment is split like an open tulip blossom, presenting the surgeon with a difficult problem.

The solution: The first step in reconstructing the bone is to join together three fragments with wire cortex sutures and then insert a transverse "set screw" to form a rigid half-tube. The wires are inserted from inside the medullary cavity without stripping the muscles from the periosteum. The fourth fragment closes the tube and can be fixed with a lag screw. Only now can standard plating be carried out. This is followed by primary skin closure over the opened anterior tibial compartment. A relieving incision is placed posteriorly over the calf and healthy calf muscles and is left open.

Fig. 34a–e. "Tulip" phenomenon. S.G., ♂, age 29, No. 75738.
a *Postinjury roentgenogram:* Severe comminuted segmental fracture of the tibia.
b *Operative technique:* The middle fragment is analogous to an open tulip blossom (*A*): The posterior and two lateral fragments are stabilized against one another using two cortex sutures (*B*), and the two lateral fragments are transfixed with a set screw to form a stable half-tube (*C*). Then the tube is closed by attaching the fourth fragment with a lag screw (*D*). The set screw can now also be converted to a lag screw to obtain a stable anatomic reduction of the middle fragment.
c *Postoperative roentgenogram:* The three main fragments are fixed with a long neutralization plate.
d *Eleven months after injury:* Problem-free fracture healing.
e *Two years and 6 months after injury:* Complete recovery

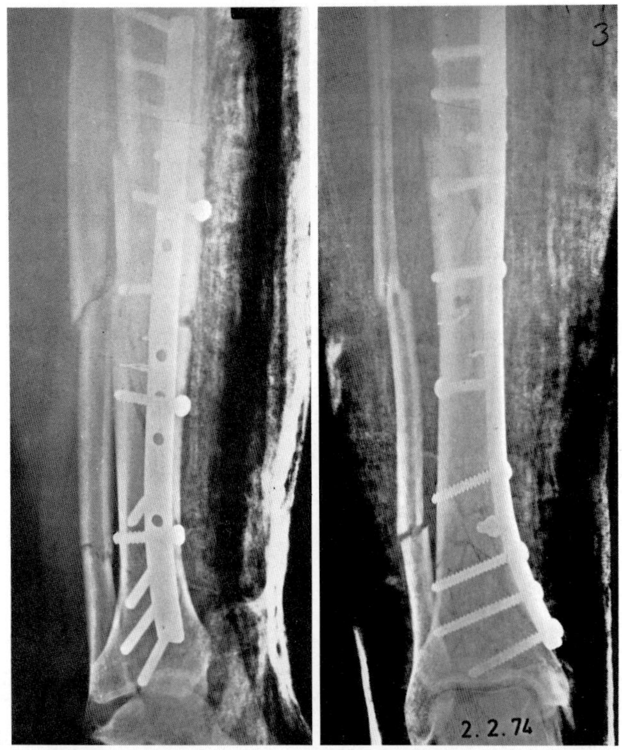

c

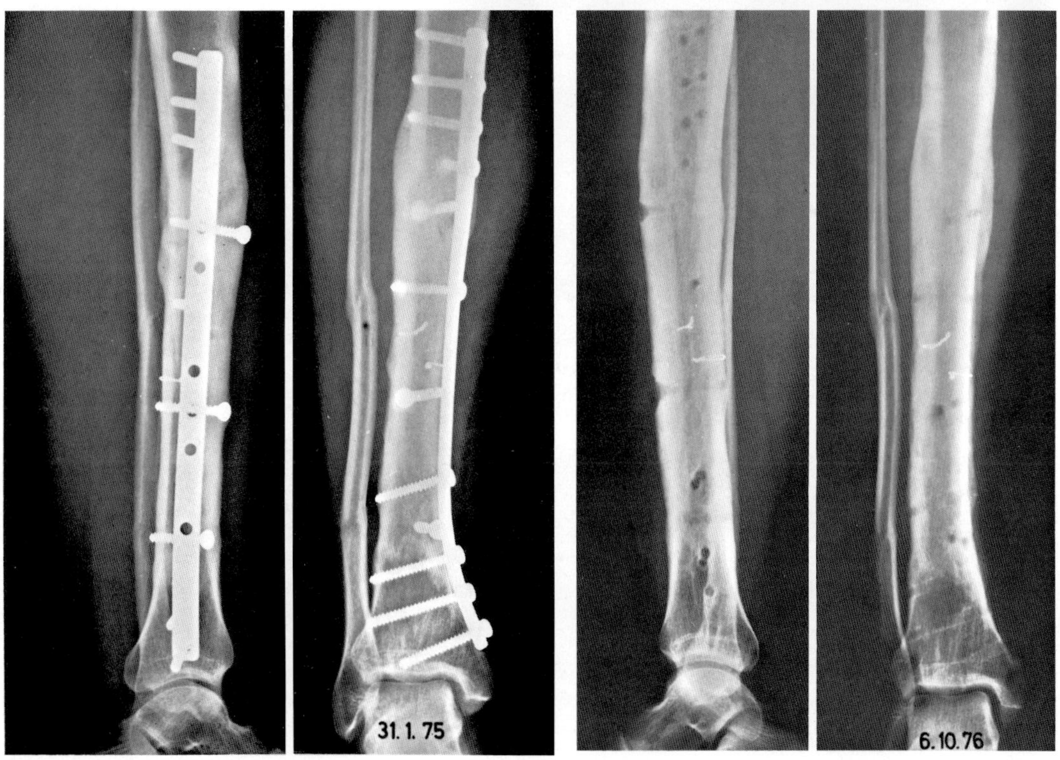

d, e

3 Combination of Wire Loop and Screw

3.1 Screw as Wire Anchoring Point

Sometimes a tension band can perform its intended biomechanical function only if it is anchored about the head of a screw. The wire is brought under tension, or its tension is augmented, by tightening the screw.

Example 1: High tibial osteotomy in varus gonarthrosis (Fig. 35)

The problem: With the medial periosteum left intact, the osteotomy is stable on exercise only if a tension-resisting element is present on the lateral side of the bone.

The solution: One possibility is that the tension band wire should engage proximally the iliotibial tract and fibular insertion of the lateral collateral ligament, and distally the head of a screw anchored securely in the tibia.

Fig. 35a–d. "Pulley effect" with a wire loop and screw.
N.K., ♀, age 72, No 131447.
a Varus gonarthrosis.
b *Operation:* Upper tibial osteotomy. A wire loop is passed proximally through the collateral ligament insertion and distally around the head of the long, obliquely inserted screw and twisted.
c The pulley effect is created by driving home the screw.
d *Four months after operation:* Osteotomy healed

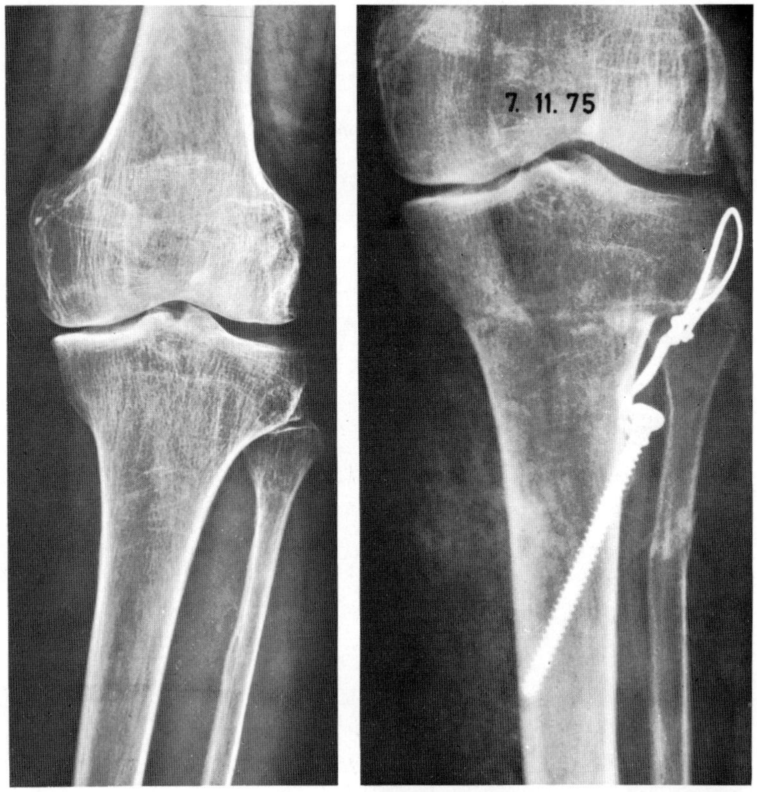

a, b

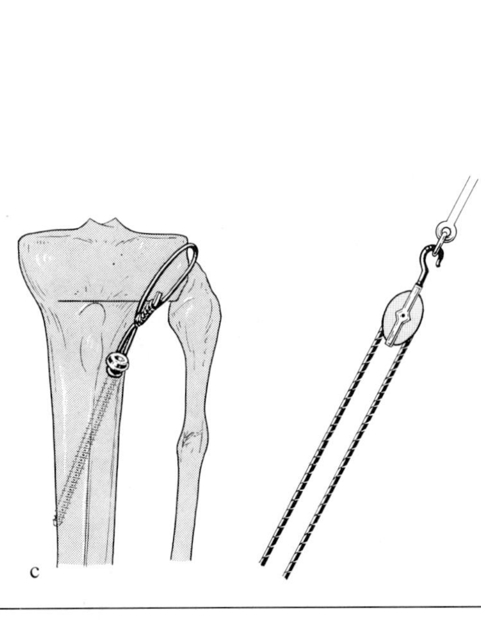

c

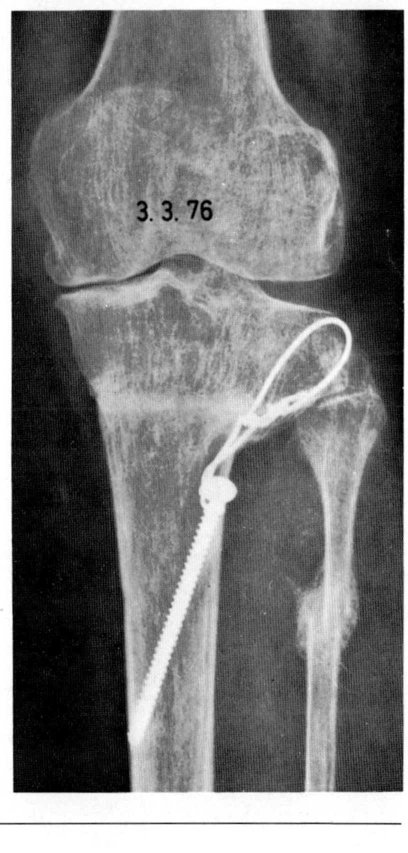

d

Example 2: Avulsion fracture of the lesser trochanter (psoas tendon avulsion) in an adolescent (Fig. 36)

The problem: Generally this fracture would heal spontaneously with bed rest and prolonged convalescence, even in cases involving marked displacement. In some cases, however, social demands (school, etc.) make operative intervention necessary in order to shorten the period of immobilization.

The solution: A tensile force is produced by means of a wire and screw, giving optimum tension resistance to the lesser trochanter fixation.

Fig. 36a–c. Exerting tension with a wire and screw.
W.G., ♀, age 13, No. 191108.
a Avulsion fracture of the lesser trochanter.
b *System:* The snared psoas tendon is brought under tension by tightening the screw at the other end of the wire.
c *Four months after operation:* Fracture healed, patient free of complaints

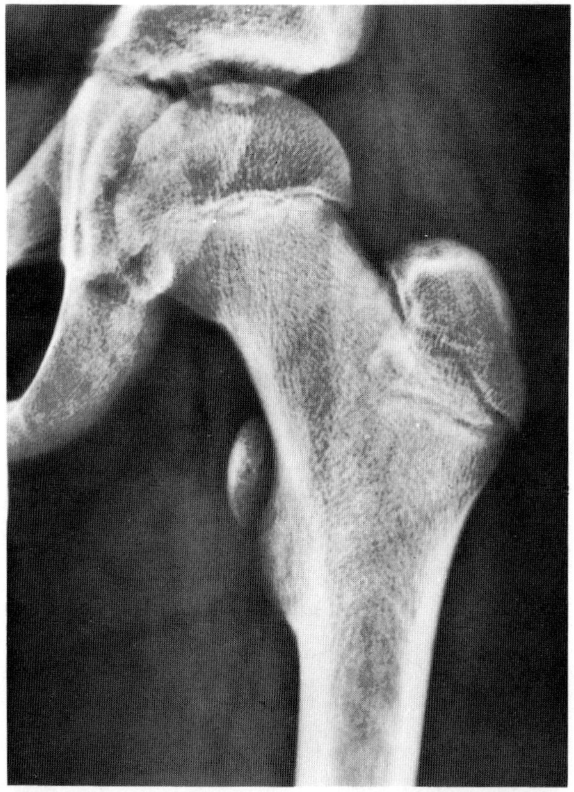

a

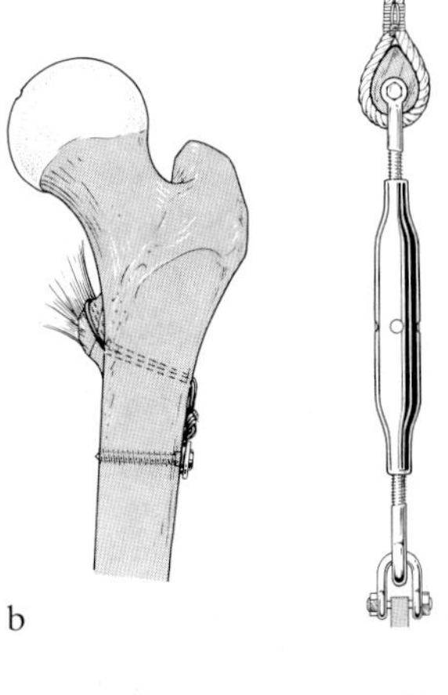

b

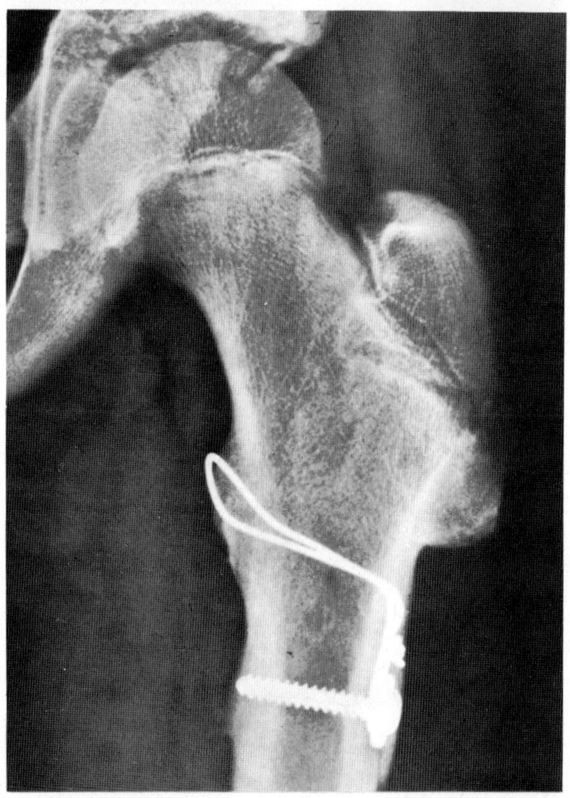

c

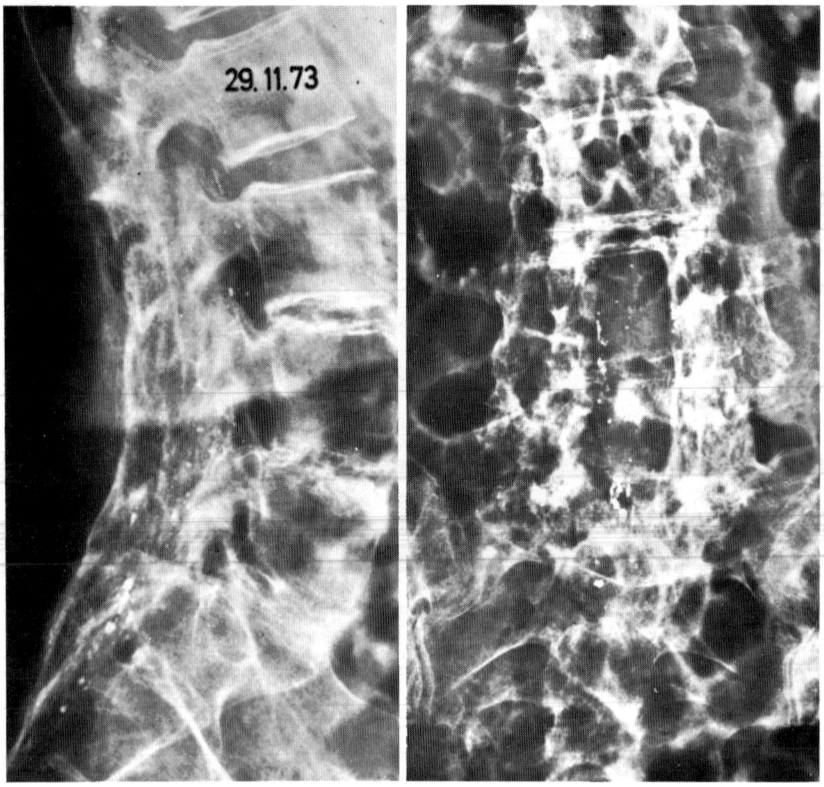

a

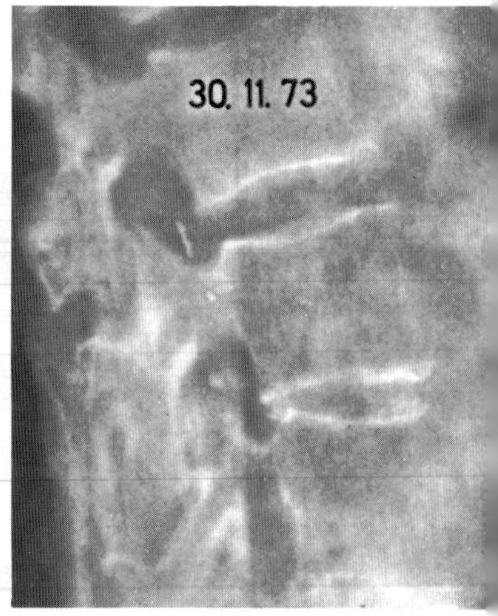

b

Example 3: Postfusion pseudarthrosis at the L_2–L_3 level (Fig. 37)

The problem: A pseudarthrosis following a posterolateral fusion can heal only if a tension-resisting dorsal element is present. If the posterior vertebral elements are deficient, as in the present example (status after extensive laminectomy from L-3 to L-5), the autologous bone graft must be protected by a tension band.

The solution: Two screws gain a secure hold in the sacrum, while the wire loop is placed proximally about the lamina of L-2. The freshened pseudarthrosis heals completely under the protection of the wire tension band.

Fig. 37 a–e. Wire and screws: stabilization of the "derrick crane."
S.G., ♀, age 59, No 139530.
a *Condition at admission:* Unstable, painful vertebral column following repeated herniated disc operations and posterior bone grafting.
b *Tomography:* Pseudarthrosis of the fusion at the L-2–L-3 level.
c *Operation:* Two screws are anchored in the sacrum and the wire tension band around the L-2 lamina; new posterolateral fusion at the L-2–L-3 level.
d The system is patterned after the derrick crane.
e *Eleven months after operation:* Pseudarthrosis healed

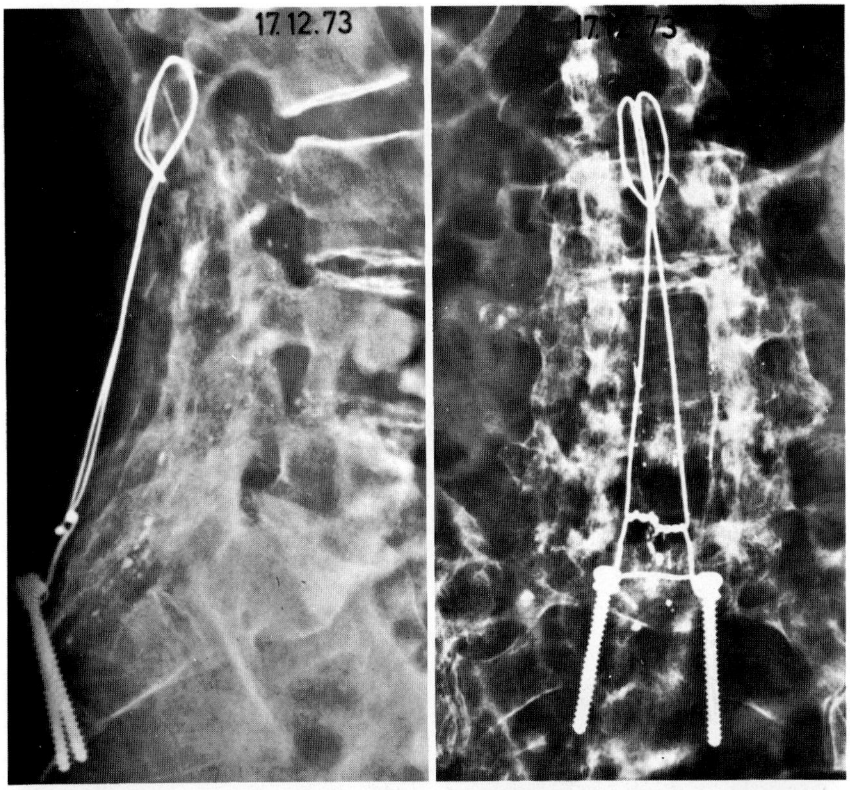

c

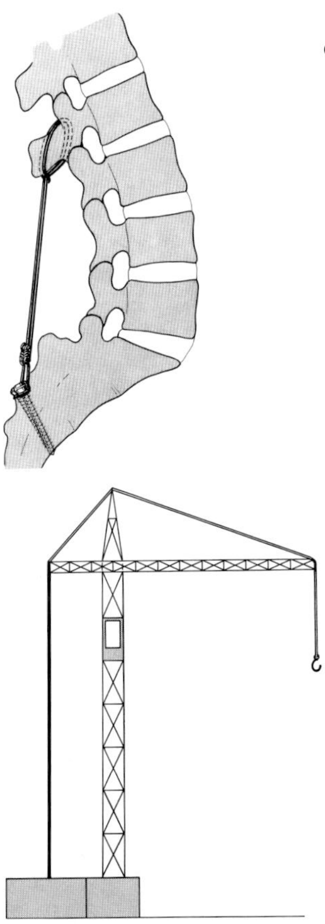

d

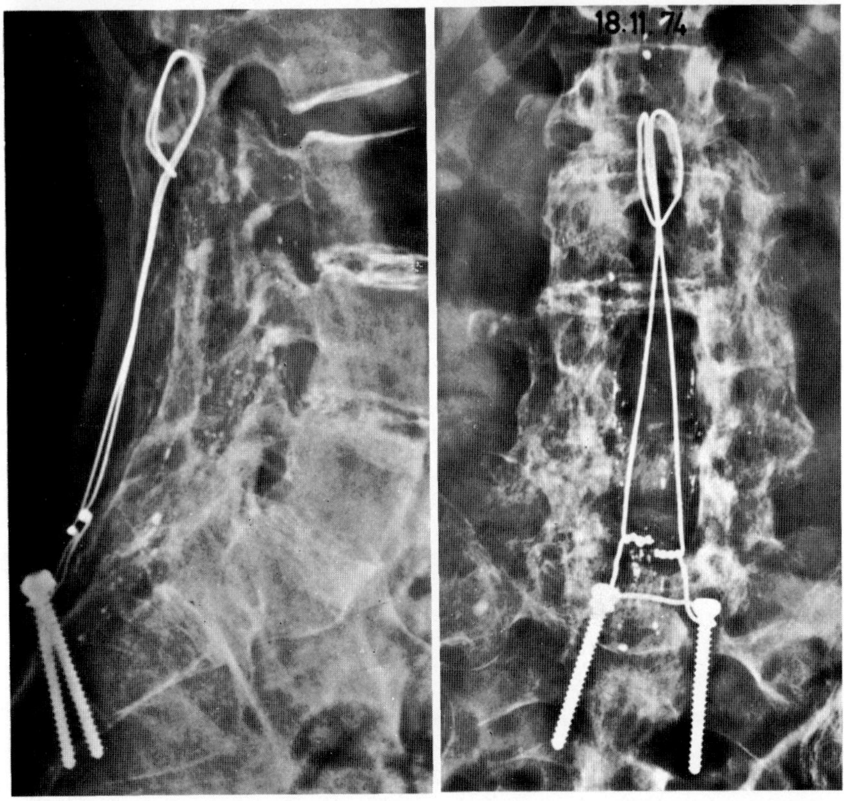

e

3.2 Lag Screw and Tension Band Wire

In this combination the screw not only serves as an anchor for the wire but also provides interfragmental compression.

Example 1: Oblique fracture of the base of the acromion (Fig. 38)

The problem: Both distracting and bending forces must be counteracted simultaneously in the fracture.

The solution: The short oblique fracture of the acromion is fixed with a lag screw inserted from the spine of the scapula. Tensile forces are neutralized by the wire tension band. The wire is fixed in a drill hole in the spina scapulae proximal to the fracture and is anchored around the screw head distal to the fracture.

Fig. 38a–d. Screw fixation and tension band wiring in acromion fracture. W.A., ♀, age 35, No. 150035.
a *Postinjury roentgenogram.*
b, c *Internal fixation:* Oblique fracture compressed with a small cortical lag screw; tension forces are neutralized by the cranially placed tension band wire. The wire is anchored on each side of the fracture by a screw head and a drill hole.
d *Four months after operation:* Complete recovery

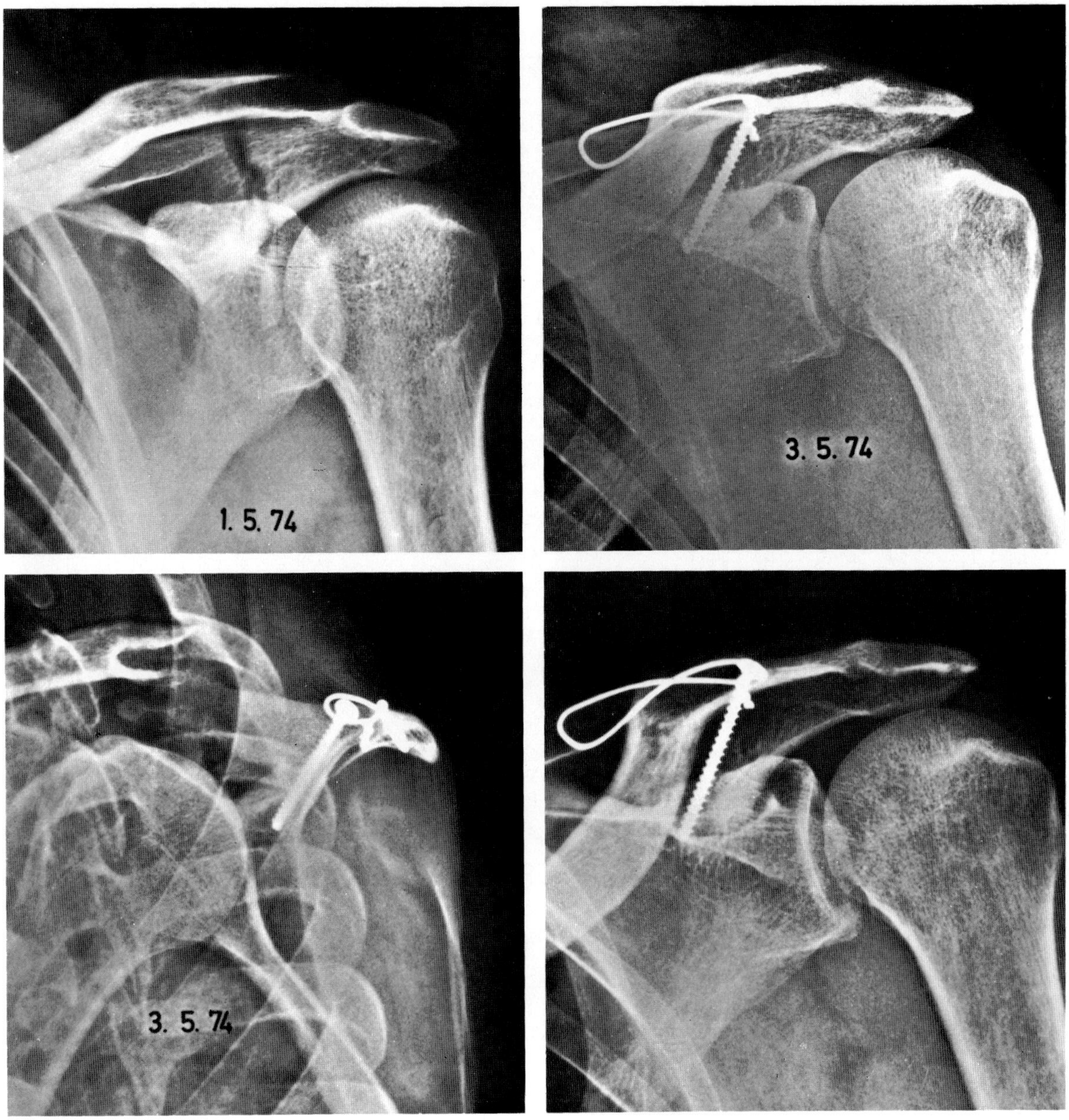

a, b

c, d

Example 2: Second-degree open fracture in a child (Fig. 39)

The problem: The fracture should be stabilized for optimum healing of soft tissues, but the internal fixation should be minimal.

The solution: The oblique fracture is stabilized with a small cortex lag screw, and the ruptured medial periosteum is replaced by a tension band in the form of a wire loop. The periosteum is still intact on the lateral side, where it exerts a stabilizing countertension.

Fig. 39 a–d. Minimal internal fixation with lag screw and wire tension band in open distal tibial fracture in a child. P.M., ♂, age 9, No. 171928.
a Second-degree open tibial fracture.
b *Operation:* Lag-screw fixation with medial wire tension band anchored around screw head and in drill hole.
c *Seven weeks after operation:* Already there is bony union, and the soft tissues have healed without complications.
d *One year after injury:* Bone and soft tissues are healed, though there is marked lengthening of the limb

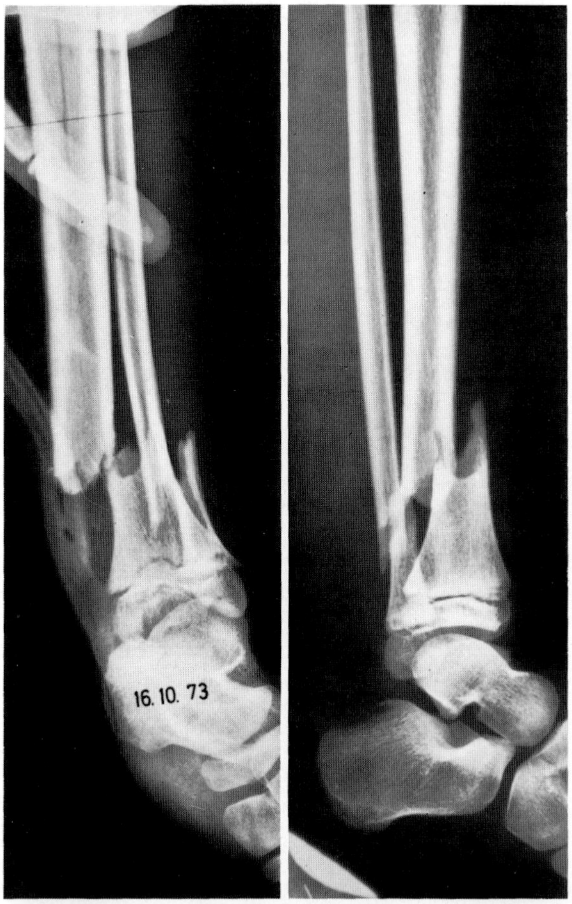

a, b

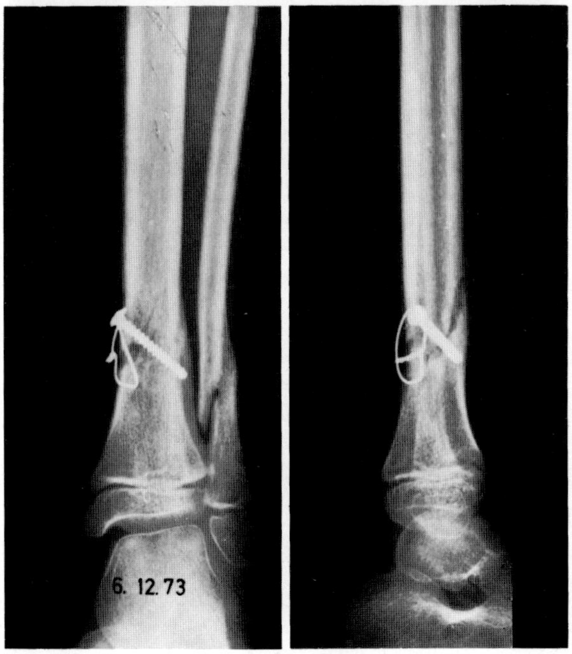

c, d

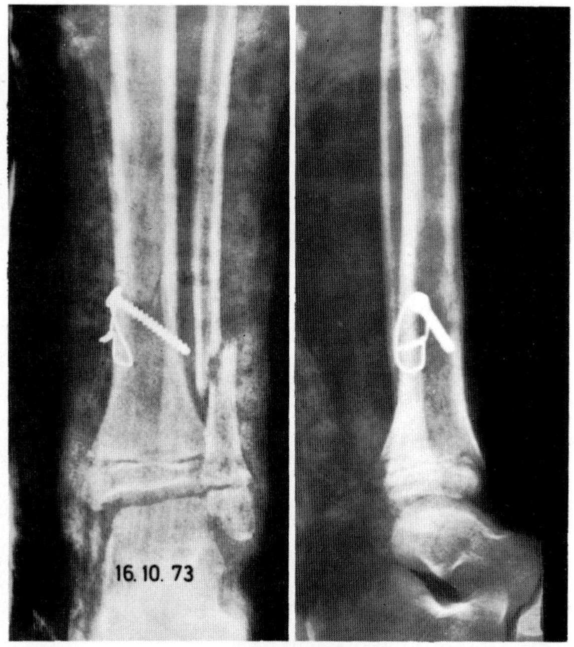

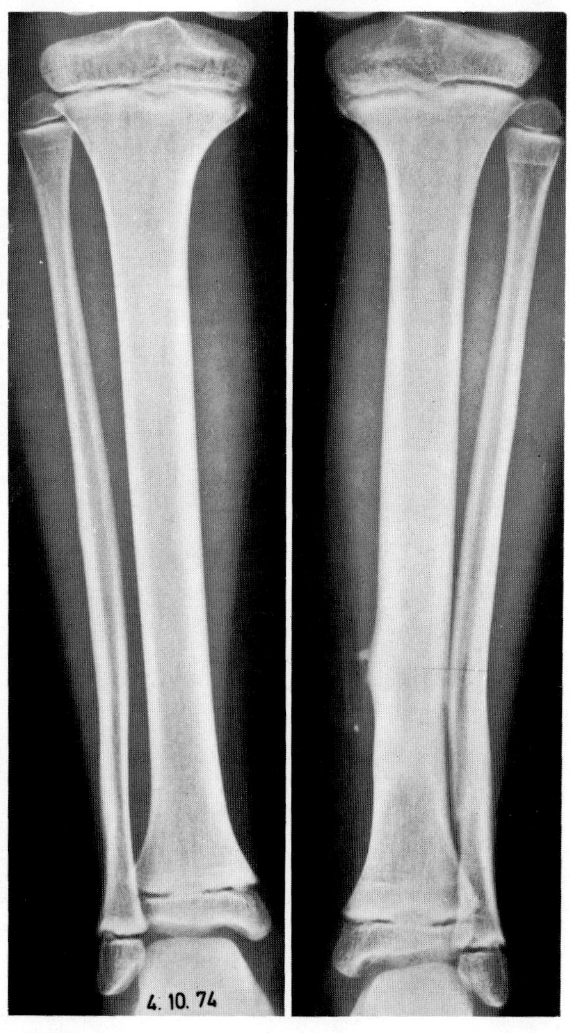

3.3 Principle of Interfragmental Compression Using Two Screws and a Wire Loop

Not infrequently, it is necessary to stabilize two fragments even though a standard plate-and-screw fixation is impossible or undesirable. This problem can be solved with two screws and a wire loop: One screw is partially driven into each fragment, each screw being angled away from the fracture line or osteotomy. A wire loop is passed around the screw heads. When the screws are driven home, the wire loop is put under tension, and interfragmental compression results (Fig. 40).

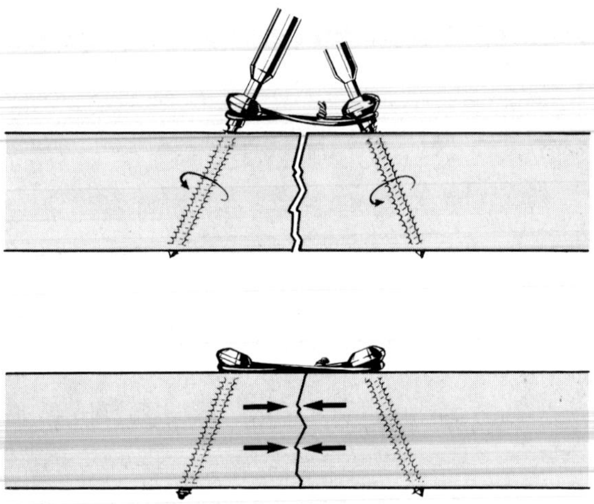

Fig. 40. Production of interfragmental compression with two screws and a wire loop.
Compression can be produced in an osteotomy or fracture by means of two diverging screws whose heads are interconnected with a wire loop. When the screws are tightened, interfragmental compression is obtained

Example 1: Compressive internal fixation in interbody spinal fusion (Fig. 41)

The problem: After an interbody fusion, the bone grafts are not always held securely in place, because the two adjacent vertebrae tend to gape anteriorly on extension of the spine.

The solution: The placement of two screws in the upper and lower vertebral bodies combined with the wire loop prevents anterior gaping and stabilizes the fusion.

Fig. 41 a–c. Compressive internal fixation with wire and screws in an interbody spinal fusion. ▷
H.M., ♀, age 31, No. 192804.
a Osteochondrosis of L-5–S-1.
b *Operation:* Compressive internal fixation in an interbody bone-graft fusion with the screw-wire system.
c *One year after operation:* Fusion consolidated

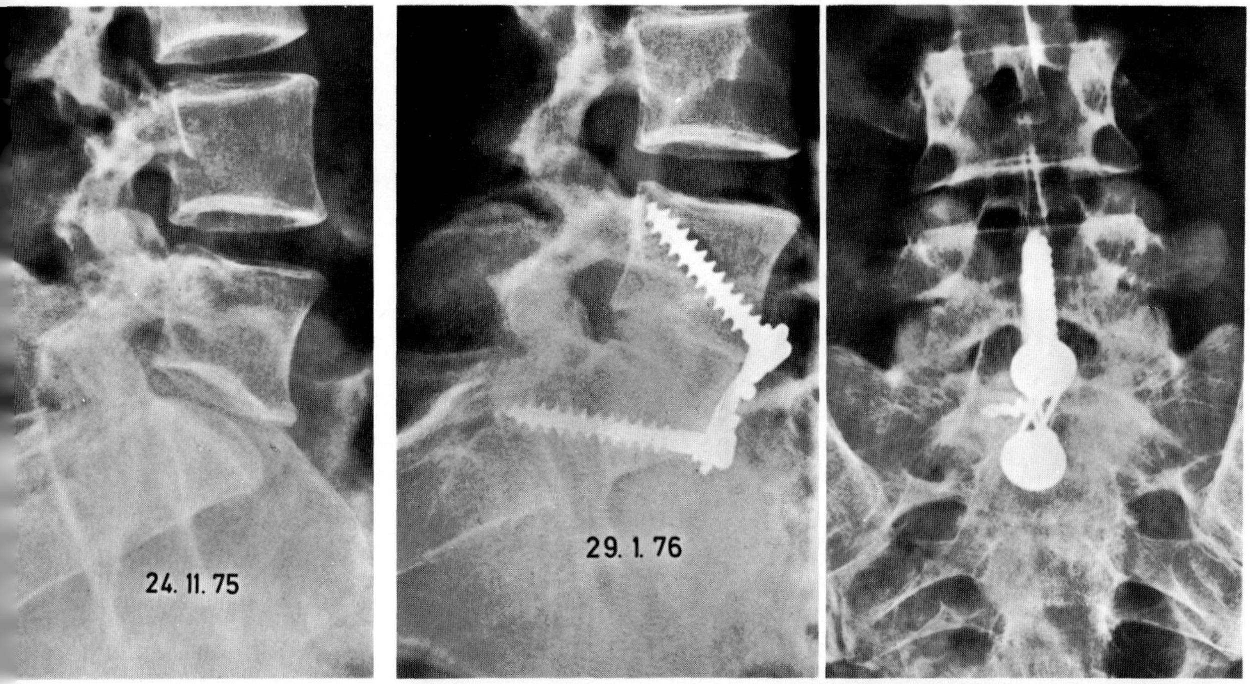

a, b

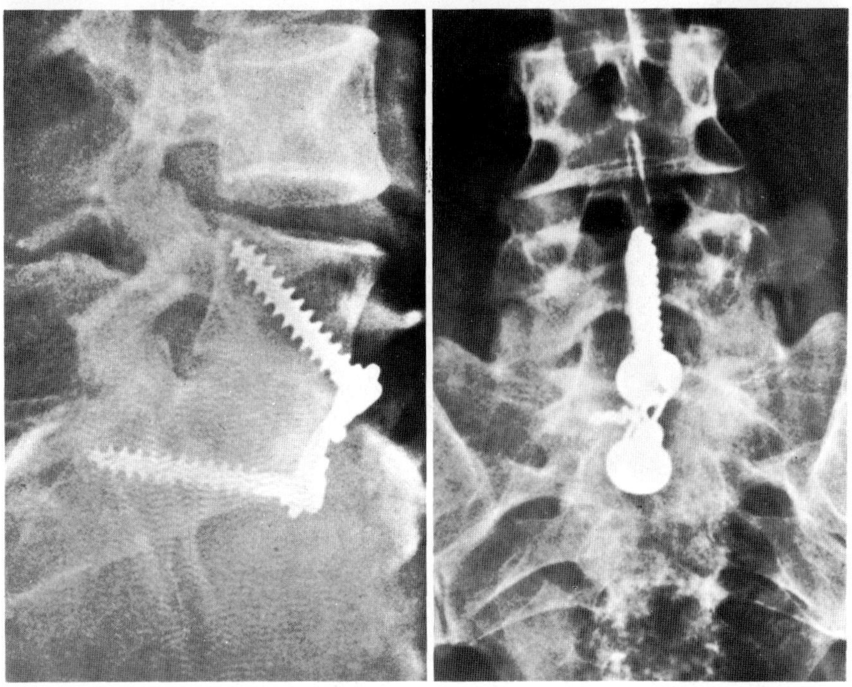

c

Example 2: Fracture of the acetabulum (Fig. 42)

The problem: With open reduction from a posterior approach, it is possible only to obtain an anatomic reduction of the "lip" fragment; the transverse fracture of the acetabular floor remains separated. An extensive exposure would be necessary for full anatomic reduction and plating.

The solution: By inserting the two divergent screws, applying the wire loop, and tightening the screws, the reduction can be completed.

Fig. 42a–e. Screw-wire technique for a transverse fracture of the acetabular floor with a complete fracture of the posterior lip.
C.D., ♂, age 34, No. 177067.
a, b The AP, ala (external oblique), and obturator (internal oblique) films show the posterior subluxation of the femoral head and the small lip fragment responsible.
c *Operation:* Posterior approach, anatomic reduction of the lip fragment, internal fixation with lag screws. The floor fracture is reduced by means of the screw-wire technique.
d *Four months after operation:* Fractures are already healed.
e *One year after injury:* Complete recovery

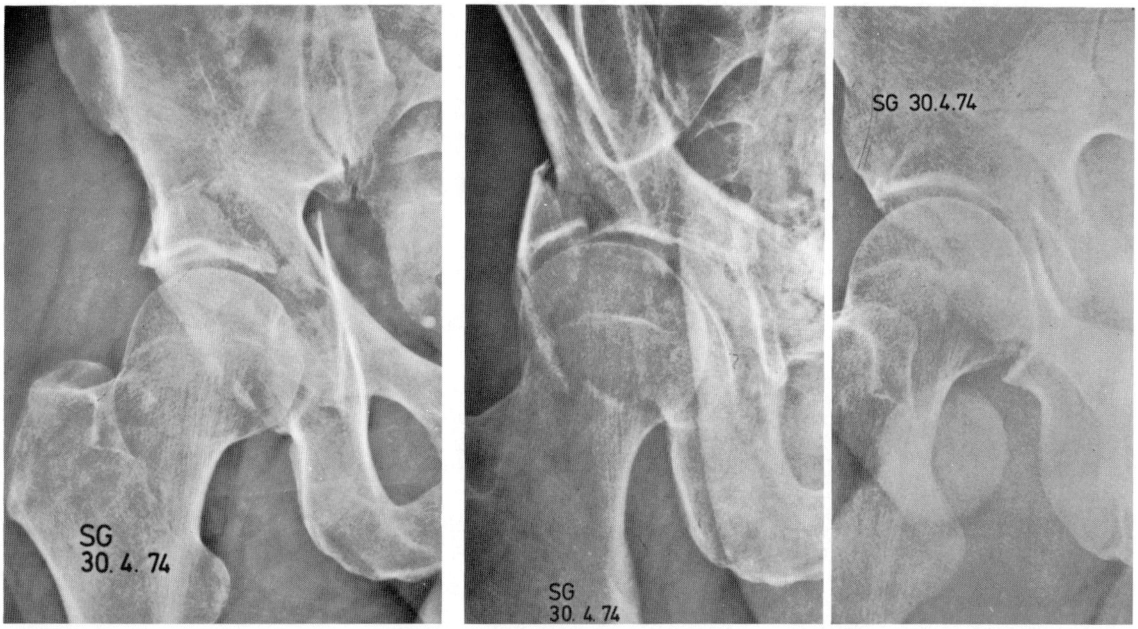

a, b

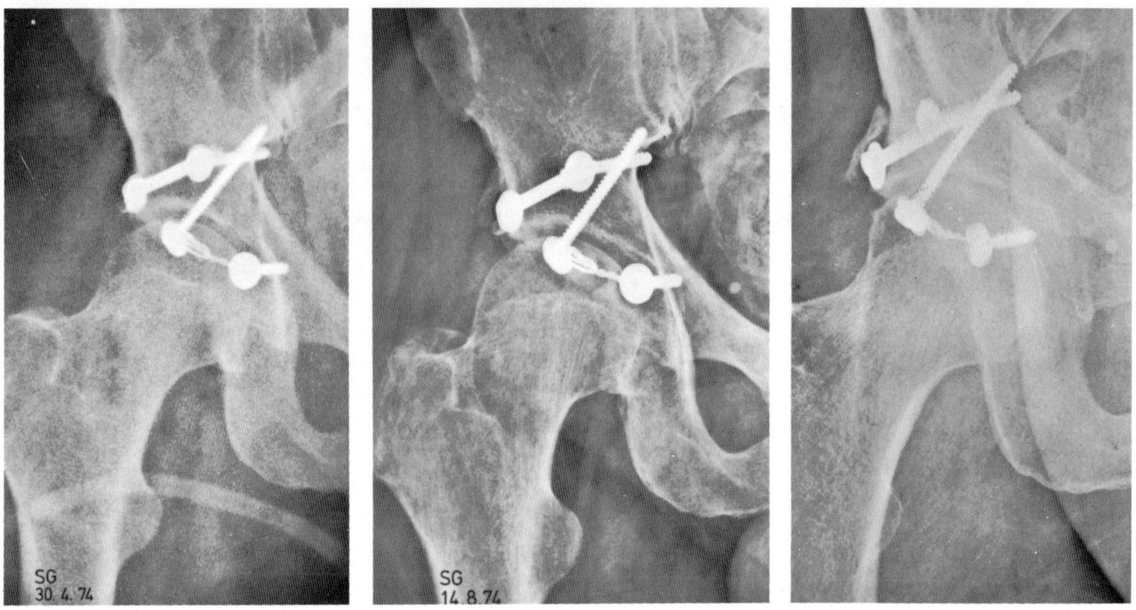

c–e

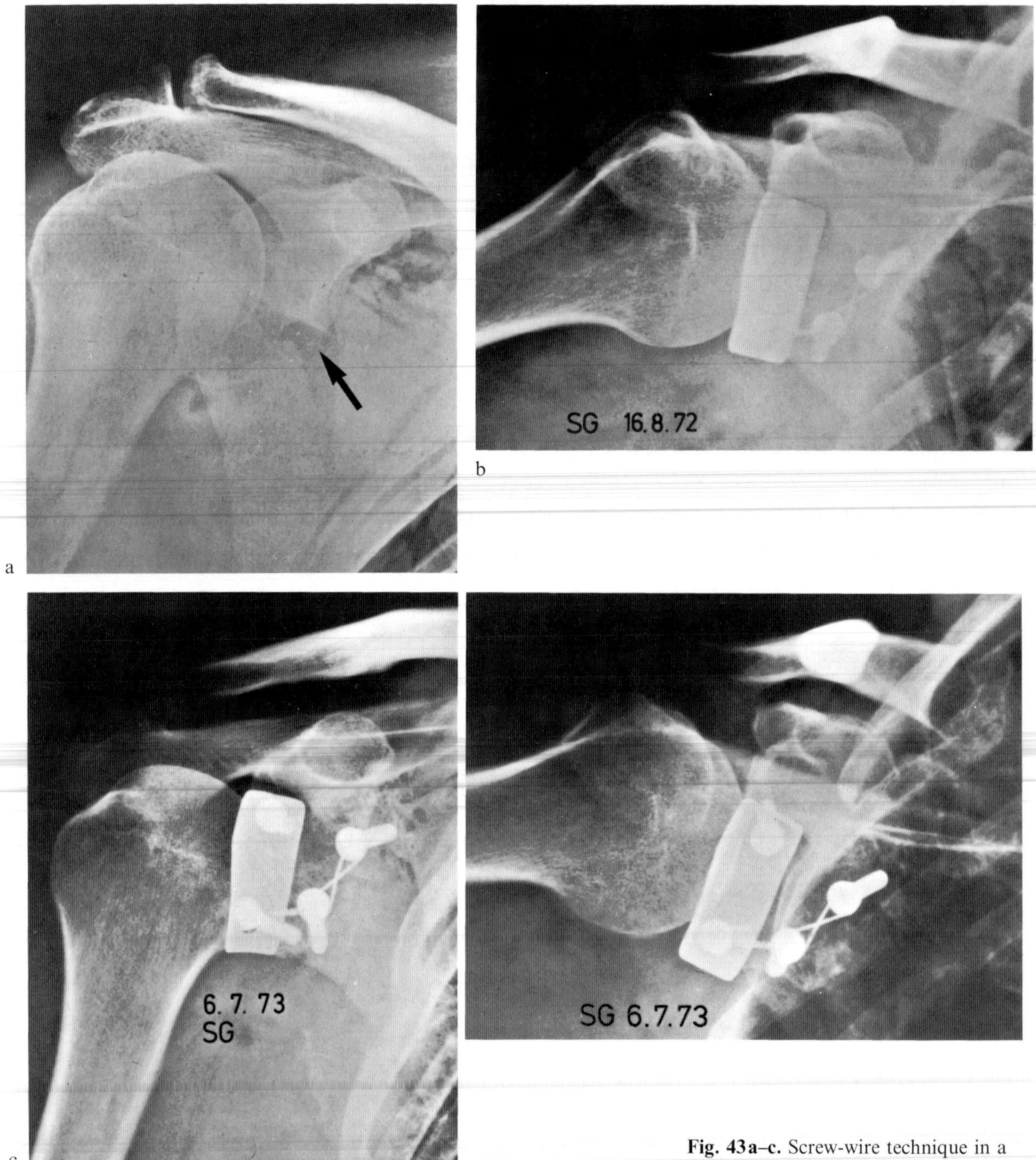

Fig. 43a–c. Screw-wire technique in a fracture of the glenoid cavity. R.G., ♂, age 65, No. 160708.
a Transverse glenoid fracture with small areas of comminution.
b *Operation:* A two-hole semitubular plate is applied from a posterior approach; additional screw-wire fixation is carried out to improve the quality and stability of the reduction.
c *Nine months after injury:* Full shoulder mobility; fractures have healed without complications

Example 3: Fracture of the scapula (Fig. 43), involving the glenoid cavity

The problem: Even after stable juxta-articular plating, the reduction is imperfect farther away from the joint. The fracture is not sufficiently stable.

The solution: The plating can be effectively augmented by the screw-wire system previously described.

3.4 Improvement of Stability of Plate Fixation by Means of Screw and Wire

In open tibial fractures it is not always possible to apply a plate at the site most favorable in biomechanical terms. In such cases there may be no tension-resisting element on the side opposite the plate.

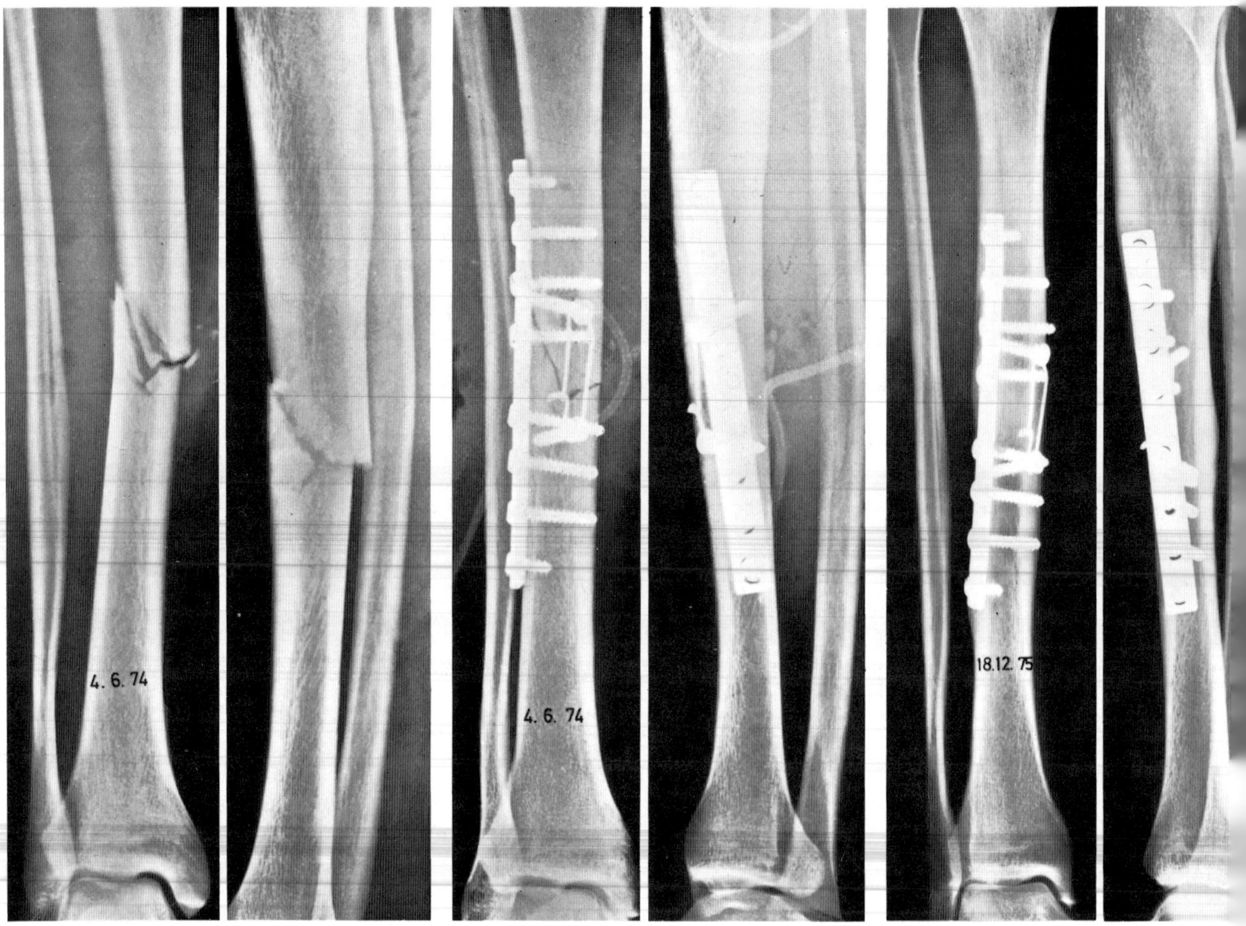

a b c

Example 1: Open tibial fracture (Fig. 44)

The problem: In tibial fractures with medial compounding, the plate must be applied to the lateral aspect of the tibia. Because small devitalized fragments are present medially, the internal fixation would not be made stable even by overbending the plate; in fact, the opposite would be true.

The solution: Two separate lag screws form the anchoring points for a wire loop. When put under tension, the wire acts as a stabilizing tension band. The internal fixation then becomes stable. Sometimes the same procedure can be carried out without the use of additional screws by employing the protruding threads of overlong screws already inserted (Fig. 45).

Fig. 44a–c. Screw-wire technique in a tibial fracture with medial compounding.
T.H., ♂, age 18, No. 177999.
a Second-degree open tibial fracture with medial skin disruption over the fracture site. Medial plating is contraindicated.
b *Operative technique:* A lateral plate is applied, and a wire-loop tension band is applied anteromedially, where the skin is still intact, to improve stability. The wire is anchored around two screws.
c *Eighteen months after injury:* Soft tissues and bone healed without complications

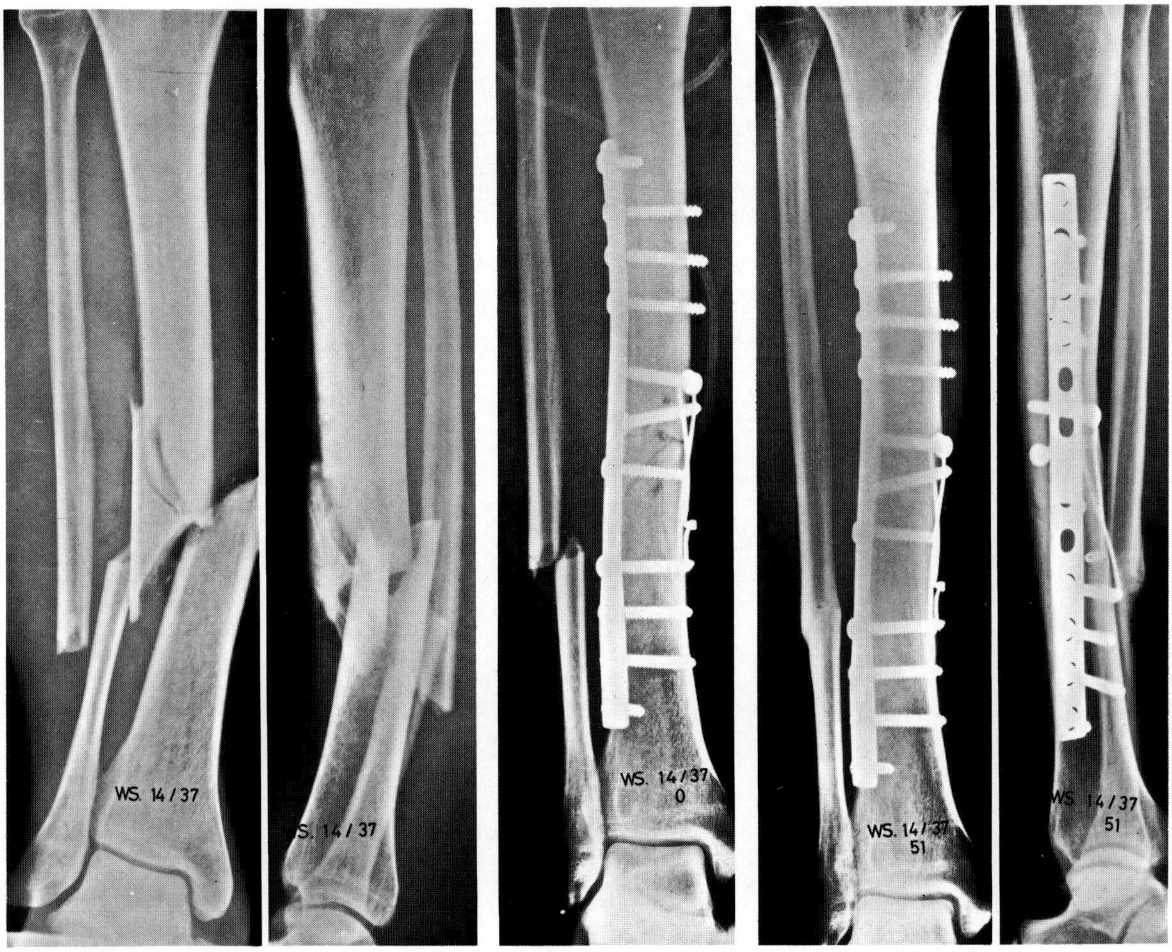

a b c

Fig. 45a–c. Screw-wire technique in a second-degree open tibial fracture. C.A., ♂, age 22, No. 180727.
a Comminuted tibial fracture with second-degree medial compounding
b *Operation:* Because of the medial skin damage, the plate is applied laterally. The burst fragment is fixed with lag screws. The wire loop is anchored around a screw head proximally and a protruding screw tip distally. By driving in the separate lag screw, the wire loop is tightened, and stability is improved.
c *One year after injury:* Complete recovery

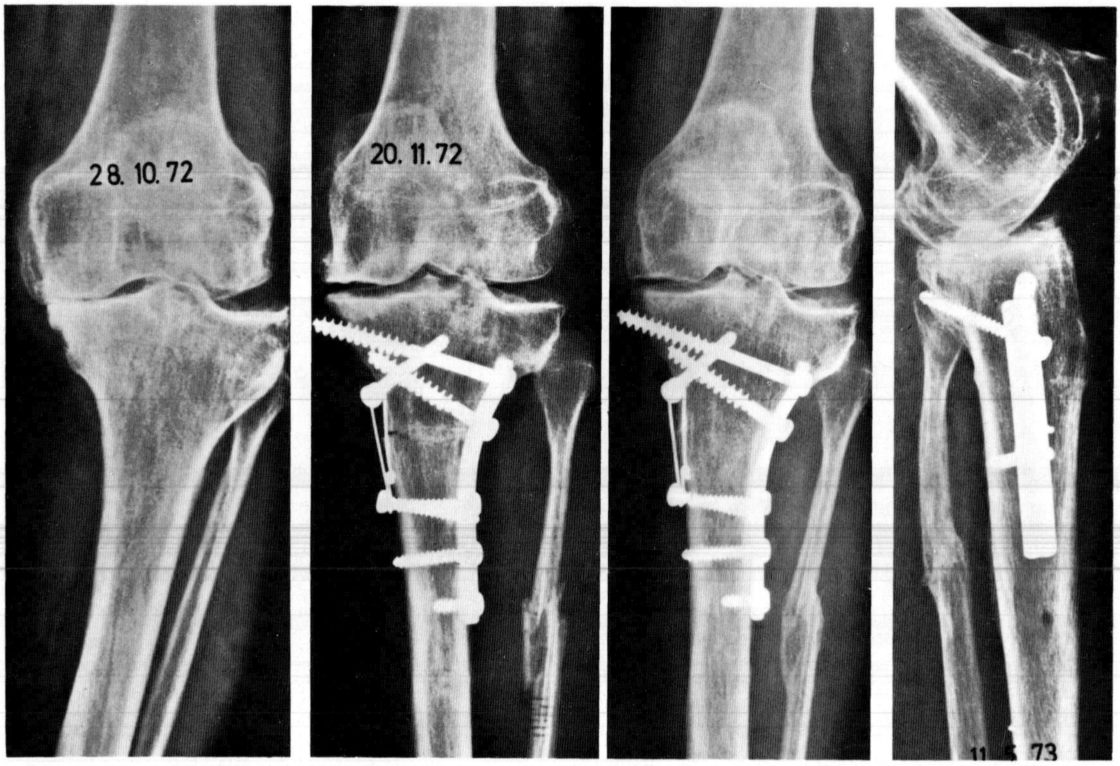

a b c

Example 2: High tibial osteotomy with medial instability (Fig. 46)

The problem: If the medial periosteum is no longer intact, the osteotomy may gape medially (since there is no tension band), leading to pseudarthrosis.

The solution: The screw-wire system replaces the ruptured medial periosteum and thus allows the lateral plate to exert its tension band function.

Fig. 46a–c. Screw-wire technique in an upper tibial osteotomy.
Z.H., ♀, age 67, No. 155760.
a Varus gonarthrosis.
b *Operation:* Valgus osteotomy of the upper tibia. A tension band is applied to prevent medial separation of the osteotomy.
c *Six months after osteotomy:* Osteotomy healed, patient free of complaints

3.5 Temporary Epiphysiodesis for the Correction of Periarticular Deformities in Children

Epiphysiodesis may be permanent (e.g., the reversed transplant procedure of Phemister), or temporary, in which case the fusion is reversible after a specified period or when the desired result is achieved.

The most common technique for temporary epiphysiodesis is the epiphyseal stapling method of Blount. One danger of this method is loosening of the staples by growth forces. This danger can be avoided by use of the screw-wire system.

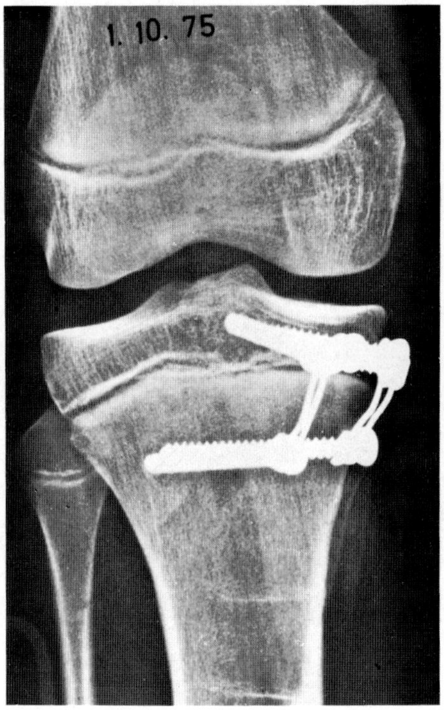

Example 1: Residual valgus angulation in an adolescent (Fig. 47)

Fig. 47. Temporary unilateral epiphyseal arrest with the screw-wire system. A.R., ♂, age 13, No. 100828.
Tibia valga following a high tibial fracture. Temporary epiphyseal arrest with the screw-wire system: Two screws each are inserted proximal and distal to the epiphyseal plate and are interconnected with a wire-loop tension band; the arrangement is analogous to Blount stapling

The problem: In post-traumatic valgus angulation of the tibia with a relative length increase, a temporary, eccentric epiphyseal arrest is indicated.

The solution: Two screws each are driven into the epiphysis and metaphysis without touching the epiphyseal plate. Growth is arrested by tightening the wire loop. When the desired correction is achieved, the temporary arrest is relieved by removal of the screws and wires.

3.6 Other Techniques Using Wire

A special implant is neither practical nor desirable for every conceivable problem in internal fixation. Using simple means, such as screws and wire, it is often possible to improvise with good effect.

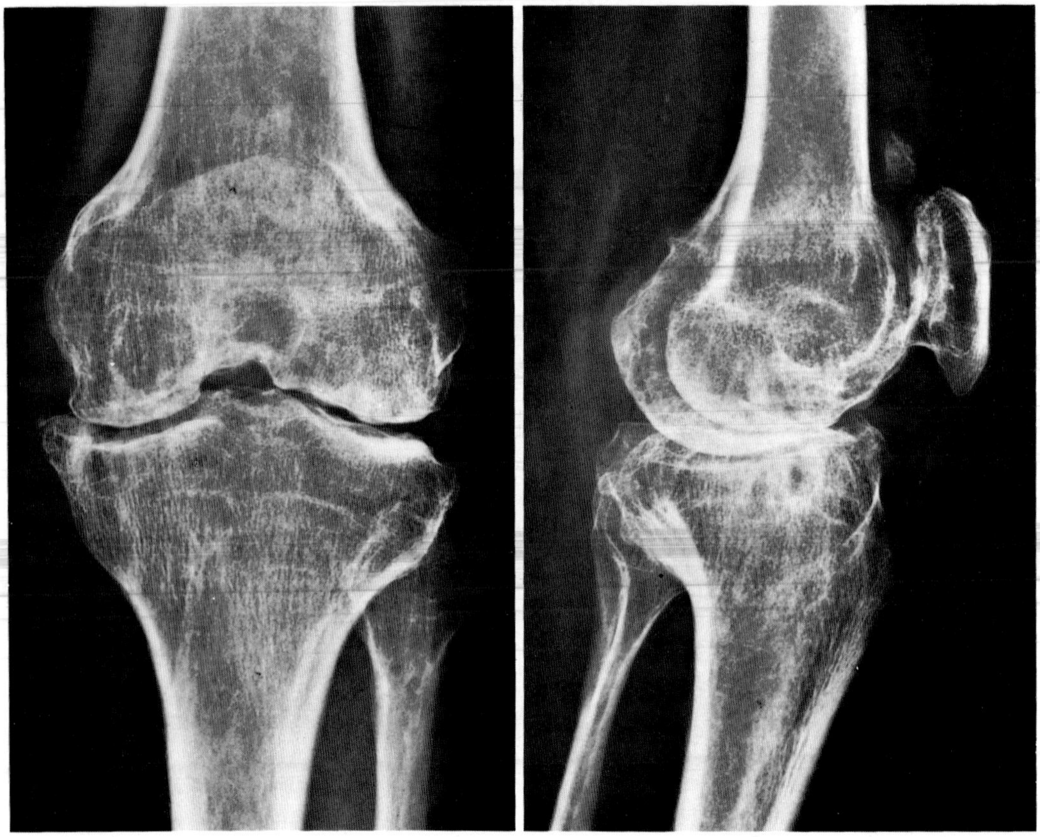

a

Example 1: Angulation osteotomy of the upper tibia (Fig. 48)

The problem: An extensor osteotomy in gonarthrosis requires a strong anterior tension band for stability, as long as the posterior cortex is only bent and so can still resist tension.

The solution: Two screws are inserted parallel to the wedge osteotomy. They must lie in the anterior half of the bone and be slightly overlong. A wire is looped around the screw heads and screw tips and drawn tight over the tuberosity to form a tension band.

Fig. 48 a–c. Screw-wire technique in an extensor osteotomy of the upper tibia. B.K., ♀, age 50, No. 203143.
a Gonarthrosis with predominant extensor deficit.
b *Operation:* A partial osteotomy is performed by removing an anterior wedge of bone and leaving the posterior cortex intact. The two overlong screws are placed anterior and parallel to the joint; the wires anchored to them function as a tension band.
c *Three months after osteotomy:* Problem-free bony union, 90° flexion, full extension, patient free from pain

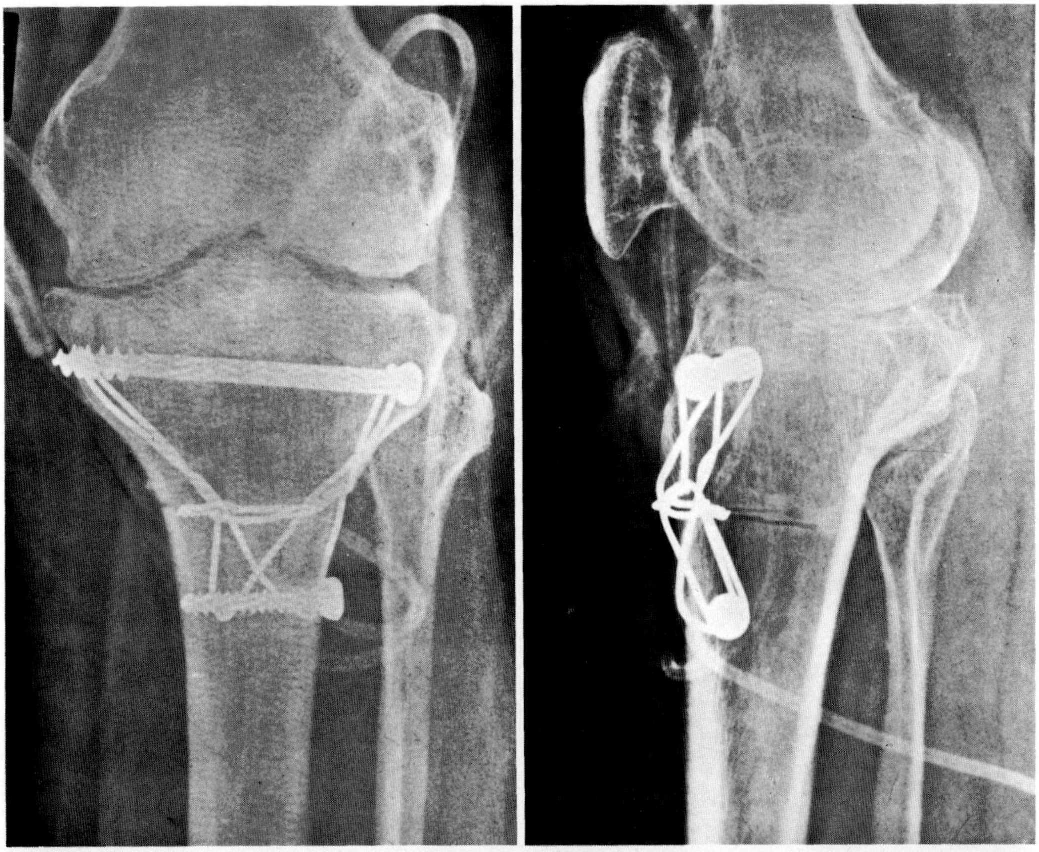

b

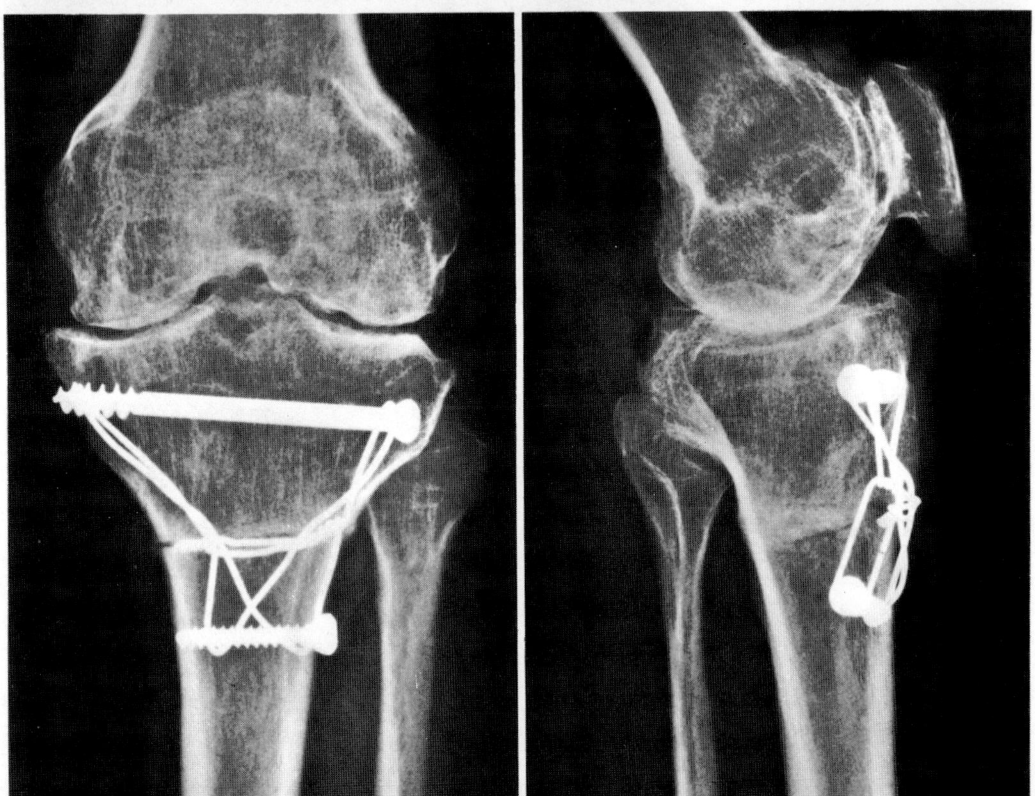

c

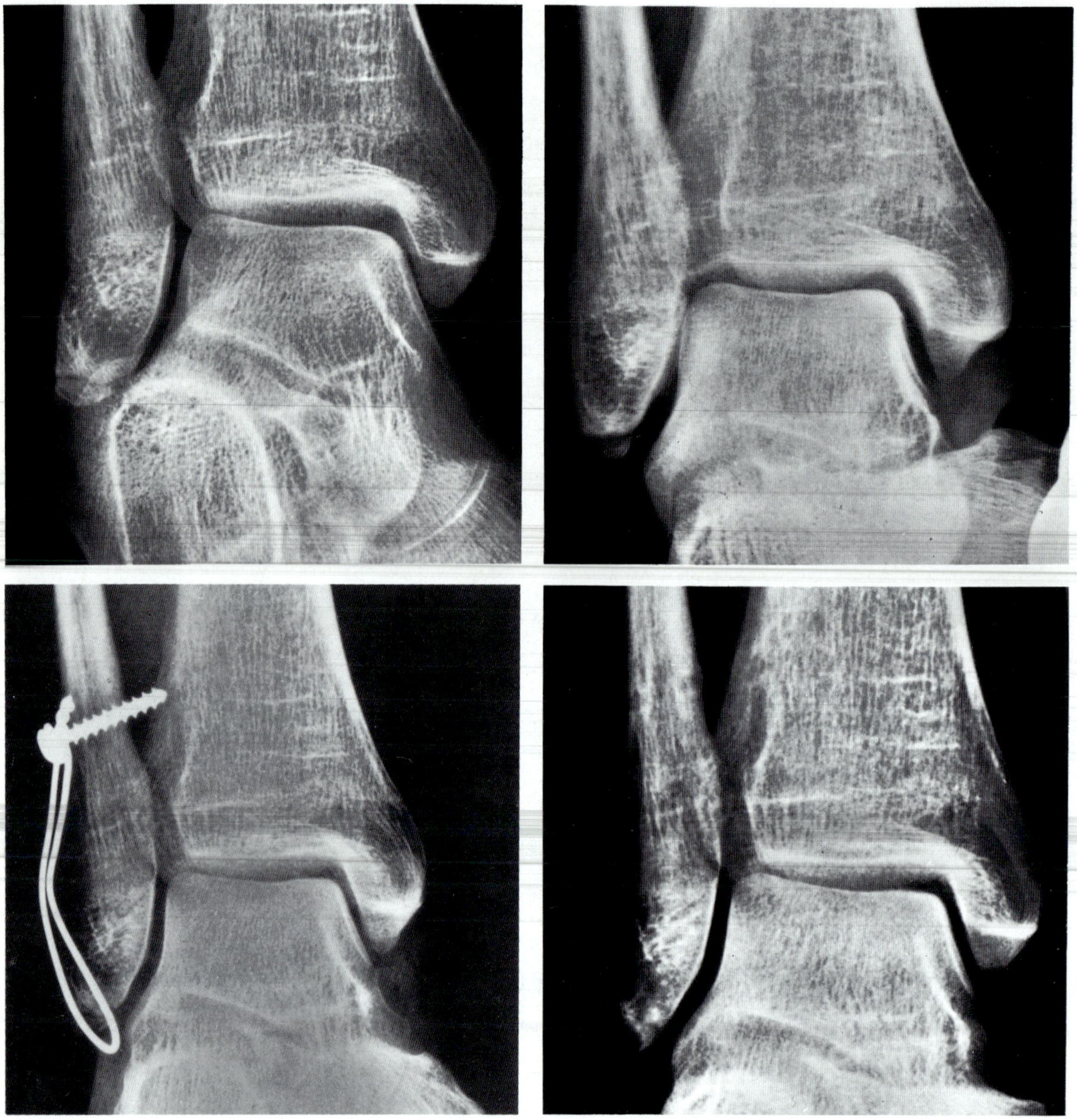

a, b

c, d

Example 2: Distal pseudarthrosis of the lateral malleolus (Fig. 49)

The problem: The fragment is too small for compressive fixation with an axial screw.

The solution: The wire loop in the tendon insertion is put under optimum tension by the screw in the fibula, i.e., the pseudarthrosis is stabilized.

Fig. 49 a–d. Wire tension band in distal pseudarthrosis of the lateral malleolus with a very small bone fragment. Z.W., ♂, age 51, No. 209141.
a Pseudarthrosis of the lateral malleolus.
b *Stress supination film:* Mobile pseudarthrosis.
c *Operation:* The small fragment is engaged with the wire loop and held rigidly in place by tension from the screw.
d *Six months after operation:* Pseudarthrosis healed, patient free of complaints.

4 Kirschner Wire

4.1 Kirschner Wiring

Generally speaking, Kirschner wiring alone does not produce a stable internal fixation and must be protected by immobilization in plaster. However, in some cases the bone fragments are so small that the Kirschner wire offers the only possible means of performing an internal fixation.

Example 1: Subcapital fracture of the basal phalanx of the big toe (Fig. 50)

The problem: Direct internal fixation with plates or screws is impossible.

The solution: Two Kirschner wires are inserted nearly parallel to each other and are bent to anchor them firmly in the collateral ligament insertions.

Fig. 50 a–d. Kirschner wire in a ligament insertion.
I.M., ♂, age 18, No. 168364.
a Transverse subcapital fracture of the basal phalanx of the big toe.
b *Operation:* The bent Kirschner wires gain a secure hold in the ligament insertions distally and in the subchondral bone layer proximally.
c *Postoperatively:* Good fracture reduction and retention.
d *One year after injury:* Fracture healed without complications, normal interphalangeal joint

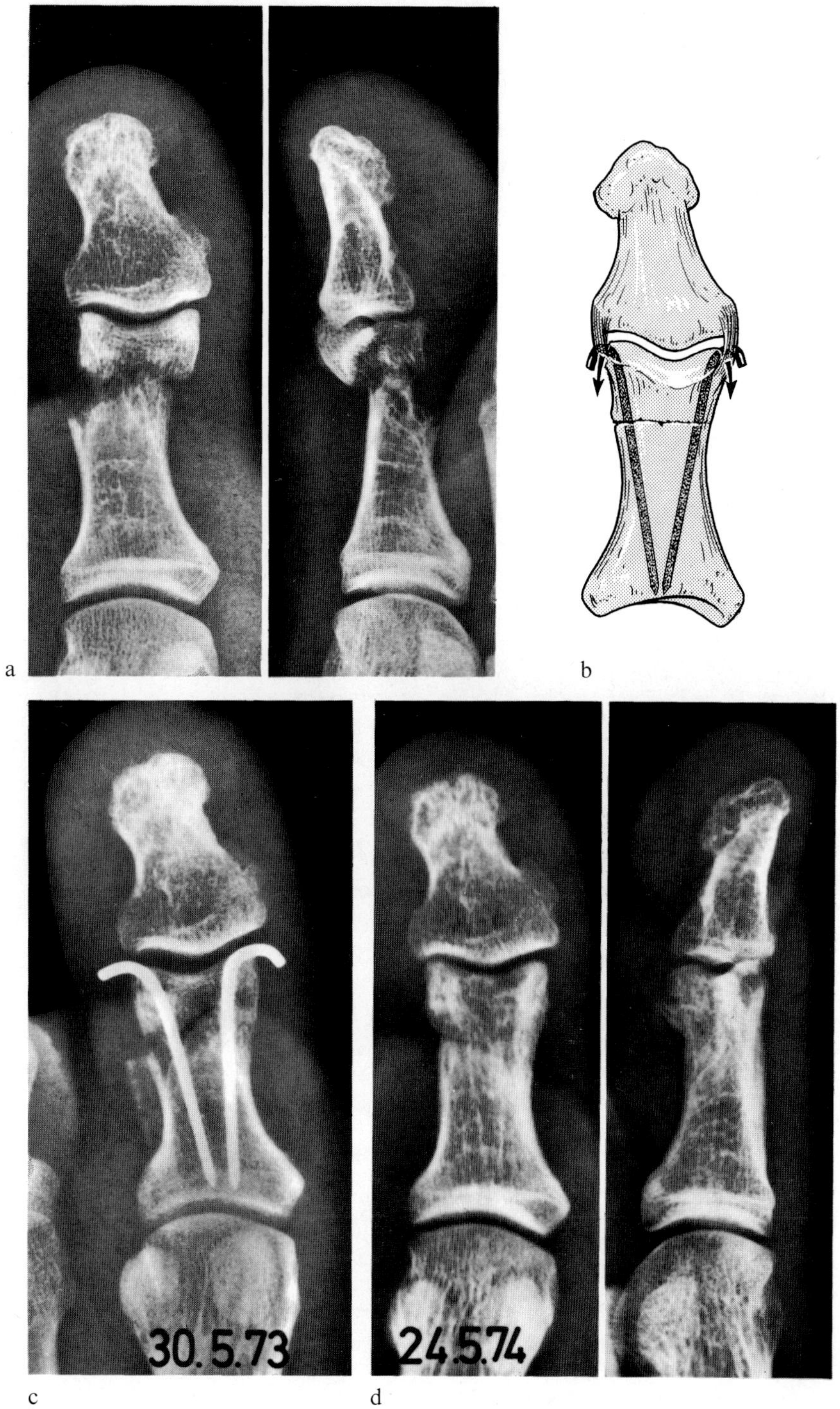
a
b
30. 5. 73
24.5.74
c
d

4.2 Relation of Kirschner Wire to Screw Head

Often the removal of implants following an internal fixation could be simplified if the various implants were easy to locate and were situated fairly close together. This condition can be met by employing a special arrangement of the screw head and Kirschner wire tip.

a, b

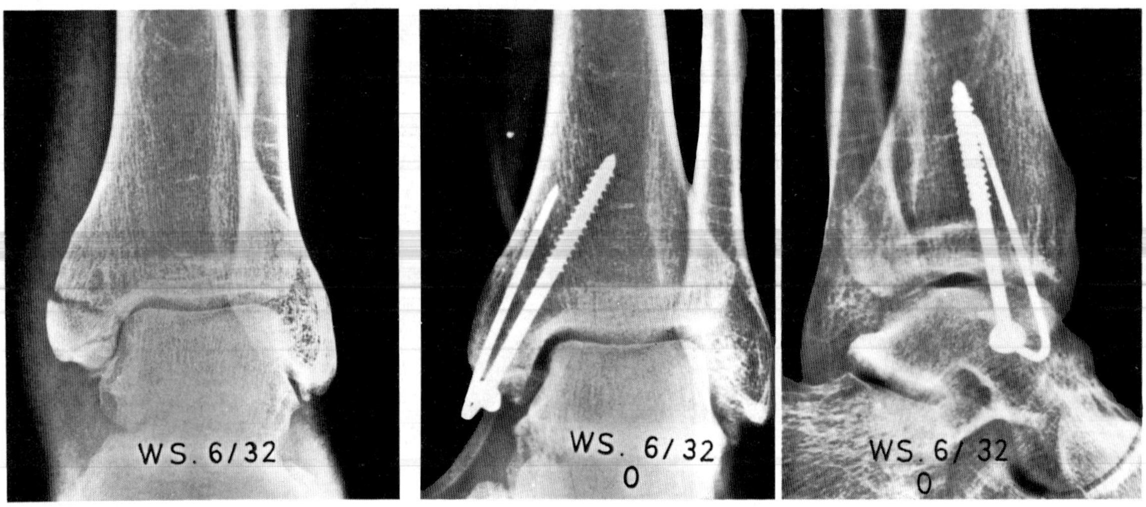

Example 1: Internal fixation of the medial malleolus (Fig. 51)

The problem: The internal fixation must meet the following requirements: neutralization of tensile and shearing forces and neutralization of torsional forces. In larger fragments, this can be accomplished by means of two screws or one screw and a wire.

The solution: The free end of the Kirschner wire is bent so that it can hook into the socket of the screw head. Since the screw is usually easy to locate, this greatly facilitates the removal of the wire and screw at a later date.

Fig. 51 a–d. Tip of Kirschner wire hooked into the screw head socket. I.J., ♂, age 19, No. 172065.
a Transverse fracture of the medial malleolus.
b *Internal fixation:* The screw produces compression, and the Kirschner wire provides rotational stability. The tip of the wire is bent and hooked into the screw head socket.
c *Four and a half months after injury:* Fracture healed.
d *Technique of implant removal:* After local anesthesia, the wire and screw are easily removed through a stab incision, since both are found at the same site

c
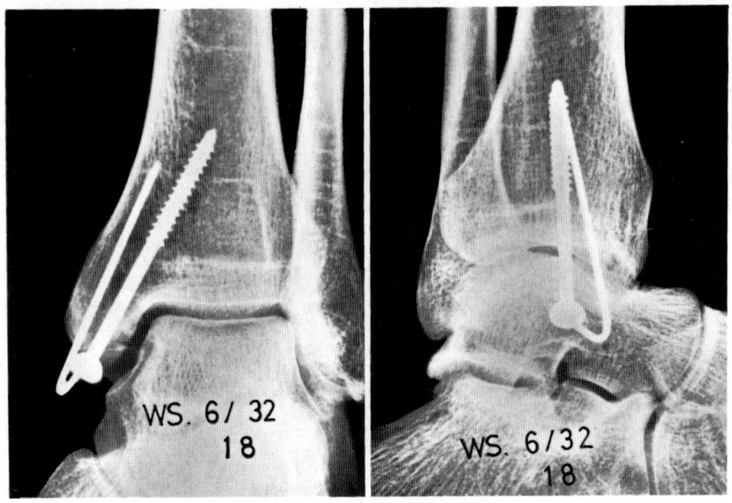

d
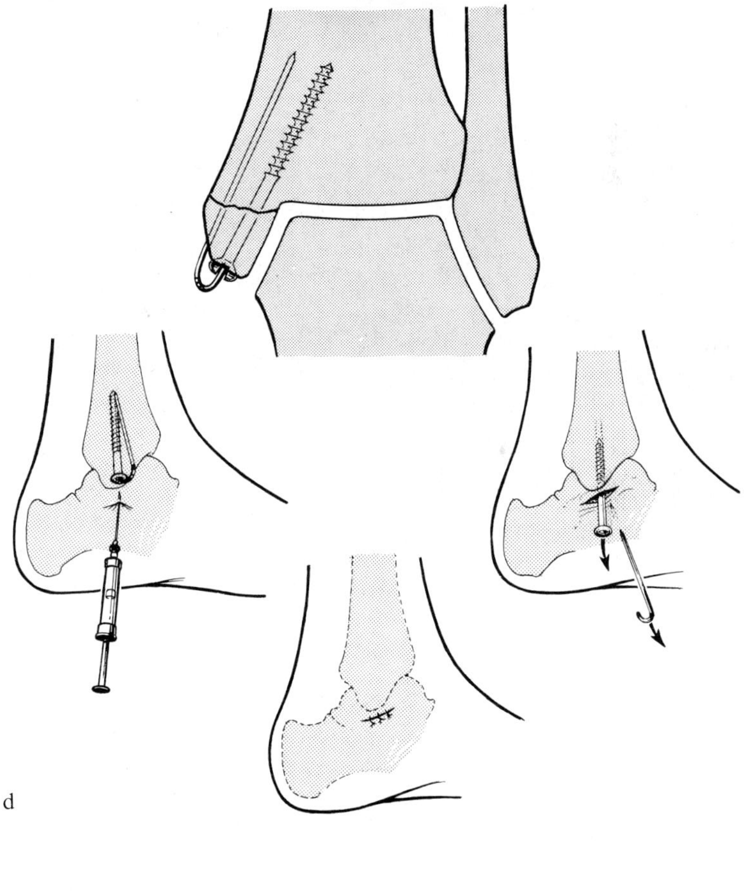

4.3 Kirschner Wire Stabilized by "Pigtailing"

Whenever a Kirschner wire crosses a joint, it has a strong tendency to migrate due to the movements in the area. In the shoulder girdle, this phenomenon has often led to serious complications. (The Swiss Accident Insurance Company SUVA has on file one mortality which resulted from migration of a Kirschner wire to the myocardium.) The wire must be inserted in such a way that migration is prevented.

a

b

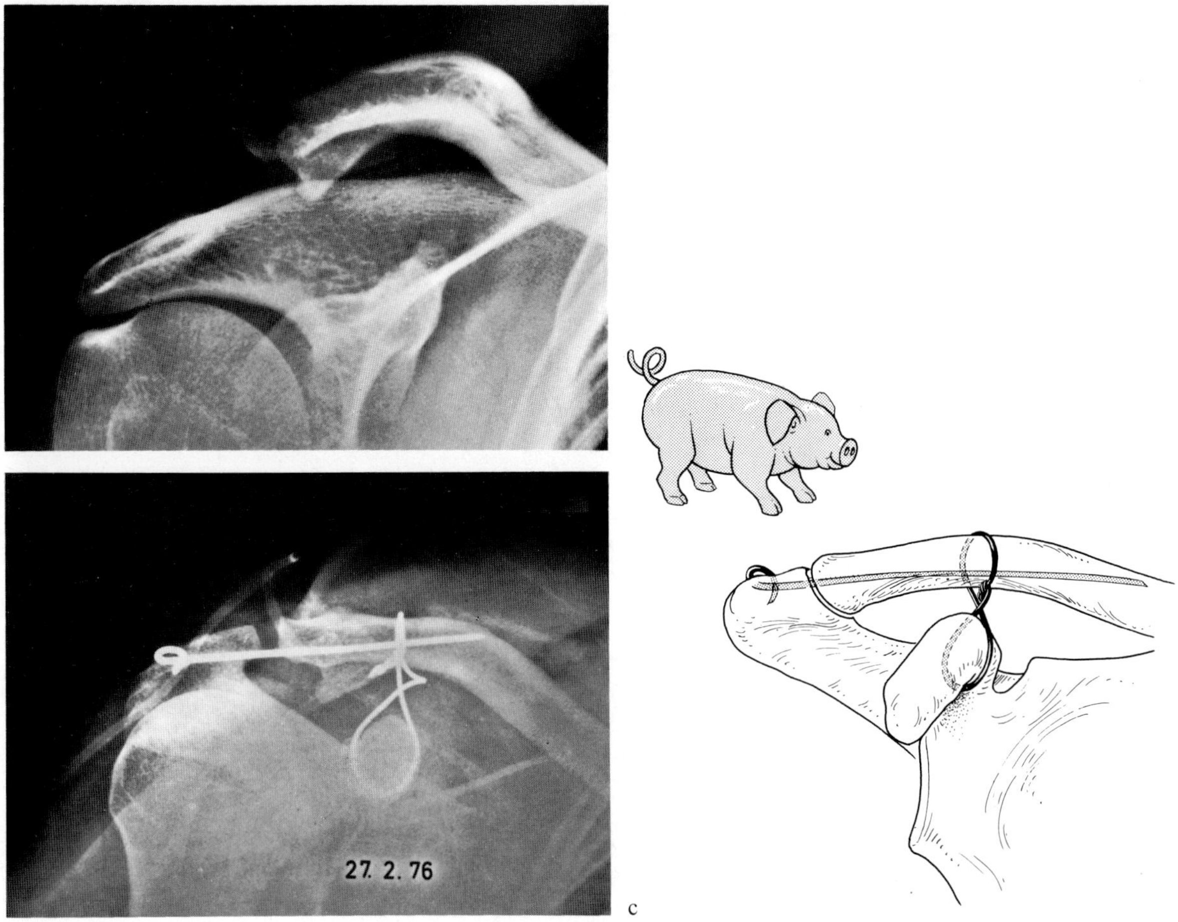

c

Fig. 52a–c. The pigtailed Kirschner wire.
S.R., ♂, age 25, No. 163472.
a Acromioclavicular dislocation.
b *Open reduction:* All ligaments are sutured. The coracoclavicular ligaments are reinforced with the wire loop, the acromioclavicular joint with an axial wire.
c Migration of the Kirschner wire is prevented by pigtailing the end

Example 1: Dislocation of the acromioclavicular joint (Fig. 52)

After open reduction, suturing of the coracoclavicular ligaments, and reinforcement of the ligament repair with a wire loop passed around the coracoid and clavicle, it is further necessary to stabilize the acromioclavicular joint.

The problem: Axial wiring gives sufficient joint stability in itself, but there remains the danger of wire migration.

The solution: The end of the Kirschner wire on the acromion is bent in the shape of a pigtail. This prevents both forward and backward movement of the wire.

5 Combination of Kirschner Wire and Wire Loop

5.1 Intertrochanteric Internal Fixation in the Child

Numerous types of internal fixation plates are recommended for the stabilization of an intertrochanteric fracture of osteotomy in the child, all of which are based on the tension band principle (angled blade plates). However, this principle can also be utilized in almost ideal fashion with Kirschner wires and wire loops.

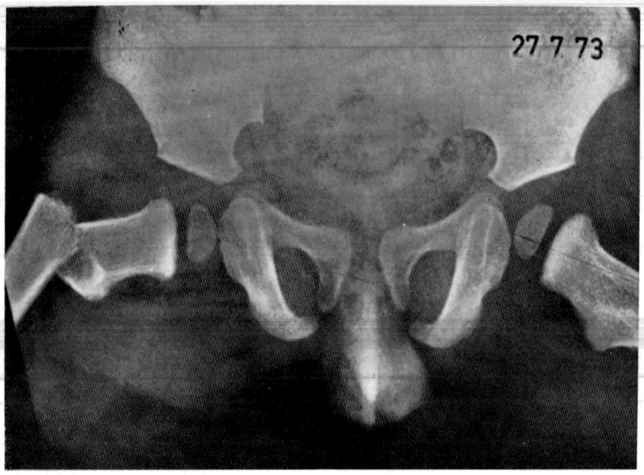

a

Example 1: Intertrochanteric fracture in a 13-month-old infant (Fig. 53)

The problem: Internal fixation in infants must be extremely stable, for remarkably powerful kicking movements can be made even in a hip spica.

The solution: After open reduction of the fracture, Kirschner wires are inserted from the greater trochanter, and a wire-loop tension band is passed through a lateral drill hole in the femur and around the hooked ends of the wires.

Fig. 53a–d. Tension band wiring of a transverse intertrochanteric femoral fracture in an infant.
H.D., ♂, age 13 months, No. AK KS.
a Multiple trauma with chest and abdominal injuries and intertrochanteric femoral fracture.
b *Internal fixation by tension band principle:* The fracture is stabilized to obviate the need for a hip spica and facilitate abdominal supervision.
c *Tension band principle:* The Kirschner wires splint the fracture, while the wire loop neutralizes the traction of the pelvitrochanterian muscles and prevents varus angulation. Only pure compression is produced in the fracture.
d *Two years after injury:* Fracture healed without complications

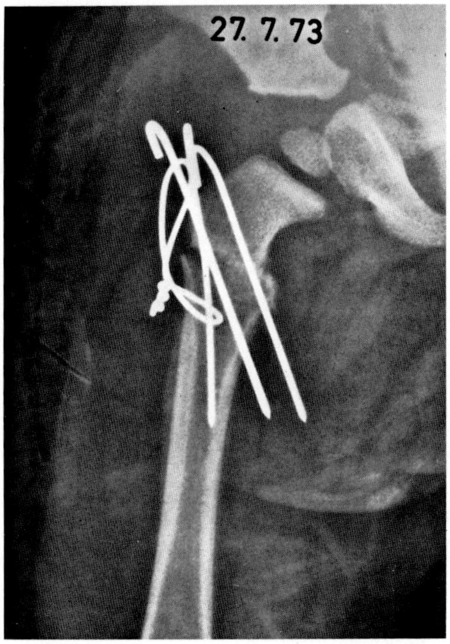

b

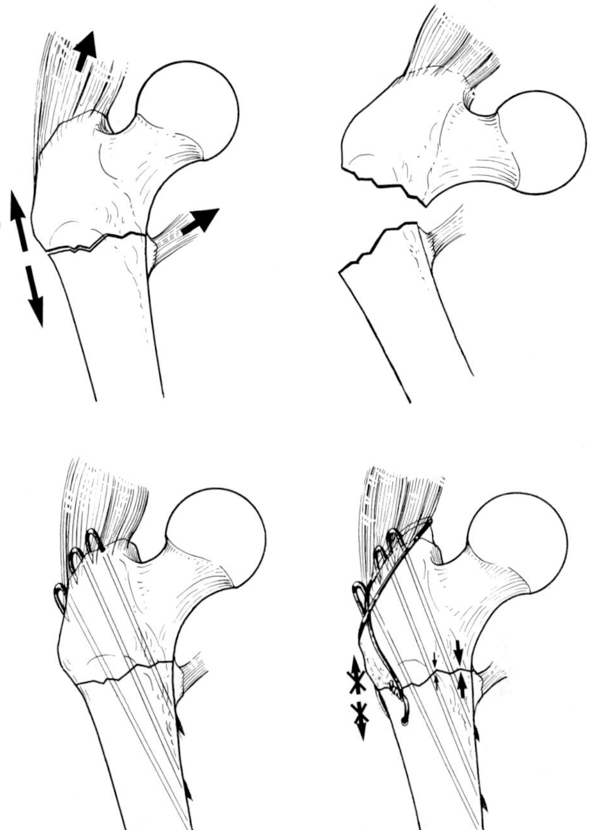

c

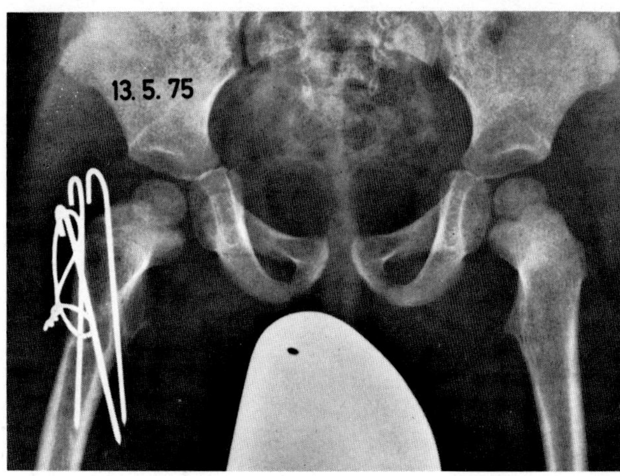

d

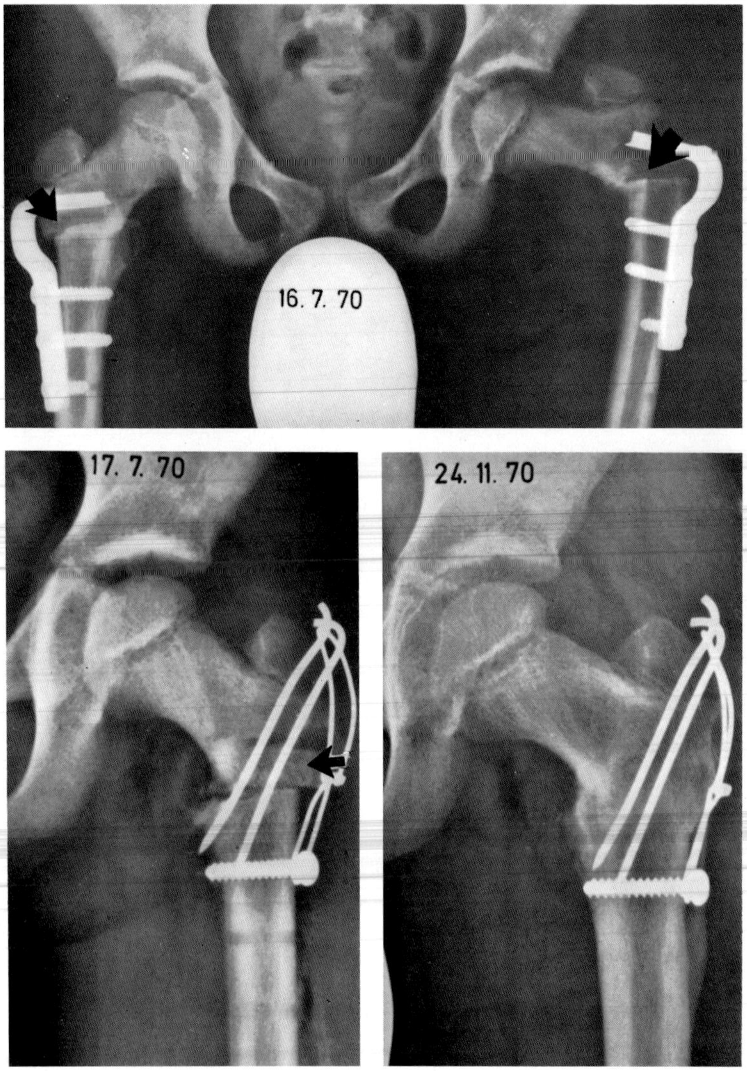

a

b, c

Fig. 54a–c. Tension band wiring after the unstable plating of an intertrochanteric osteotomy in a child.
L.N., ♂, age 9, No. 90855.
a *Postoperative instability:* The stress-bearing bony bridge between the plate blade and osteotomy has broken free.
b *Operation:* Reduction with the plate in situ. Transfixation of the two fragments with two Kirschner wires. Plate removal and application of wire tension band around the Kirschner wires and screw head. The bone fragment is held in place by compression.
c *Four months after reoperation:* Osteotomy healed without complications

Example 2: Unstable plating of an intertrochanteric osteotomy in a child (Fig. 54)

The problem: The all-important bony bridge between the plate blade and osteotomy has broken free, requiring that a different technique be used at reoperation.

The solution: After open reduction of the osteotomy with the plate in situ, Kirschner wires are inserted and the plate is then removed. A wire loop is passed around the Kirschner wires and proximal screw to serve as a tension band. The broken fragment is held securely in place.

5.2 Kirschner Wires and Wire Loop Performing the Function of an Angled Blade Plate

When operating on the proximal femur in the child, it is possible to fashion a "tailor-made" angled blade plate intraoperatively from Kirschner wires.

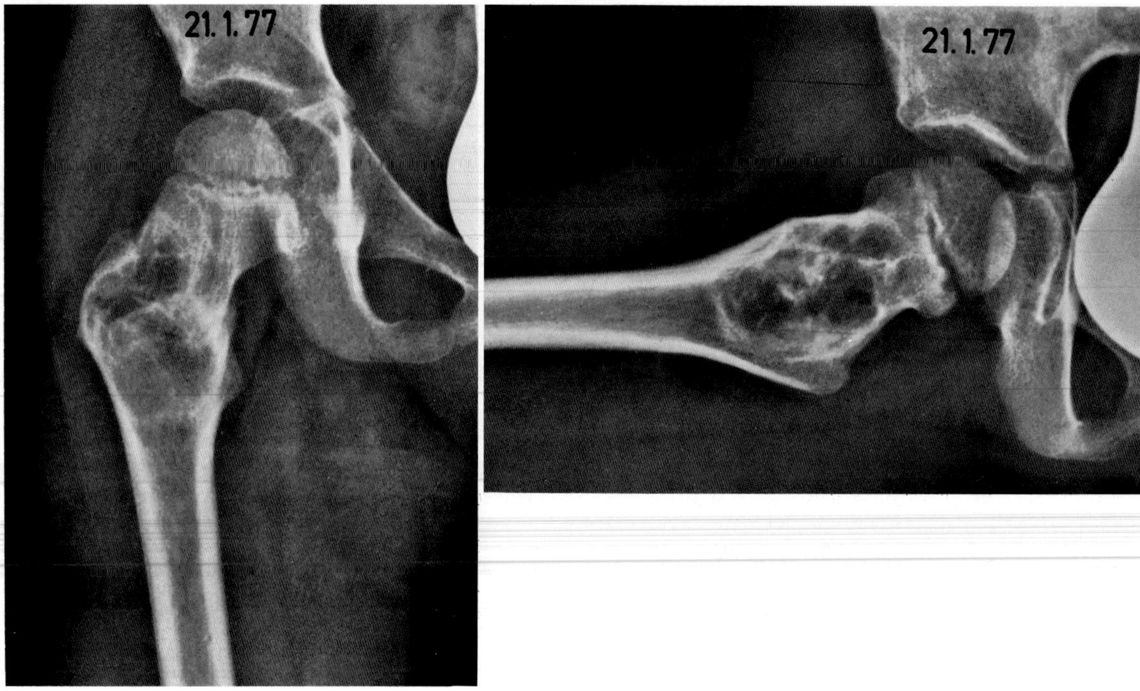

a

Example 1: Bone grafting and internal splinting after the excision of a cystic tumor from the intertrochanteric area (Fig. 55)

The problem: After radical excision of the tumor, the femoral neck remains profoundly weakened, with a risk of fracture despite adequate grafting with autologous cancellous bone.

The solution: Three 3-mm-thick Kirschner wires are inserted along the femoral neck axis until they enter the epiphyseal plate, so that the femoral neck is securely splinted. The bending strength of the intertrochanteric area is enhanced by angling the three wires and attaching them under tension to the femoral shaft by two wire loops.

Fig. 55a–e. Splinting of the femoral neck with Kirschner wires in a child. B.M., ♀, age 9, No. 204636.
a Osteofibroma with weakening of the femoral neck.
b *Operation:* Excision of tumor, cancellous bone grafting. The weakened femoral neck is splinted internally with two thick Kirschner wires. The angled wires are stabilized against the femoral shaft with two wire loops.
c *Schematic:* The internal splinting corresponds to that of a 130° angled blade plate. The loops prevent migration of the Kirschner wires.
d *Two months after operation:* Complete healing of cancellous bone.
e *Nineteen months after operation:* No tumor recurrence, femoral neck normal

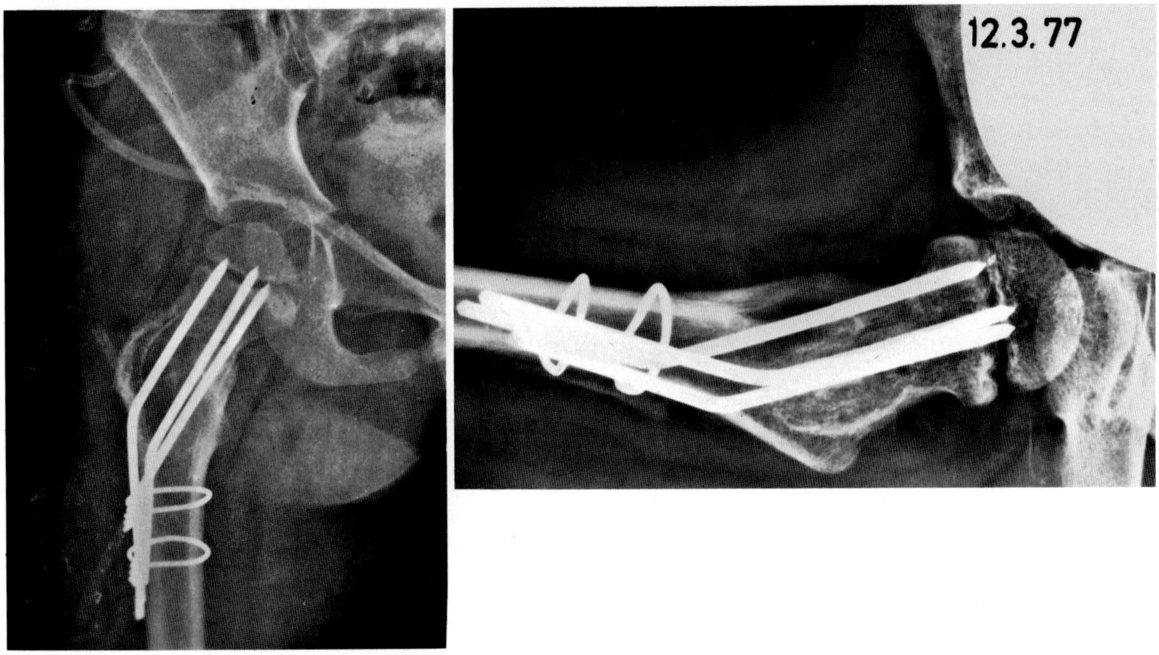

b

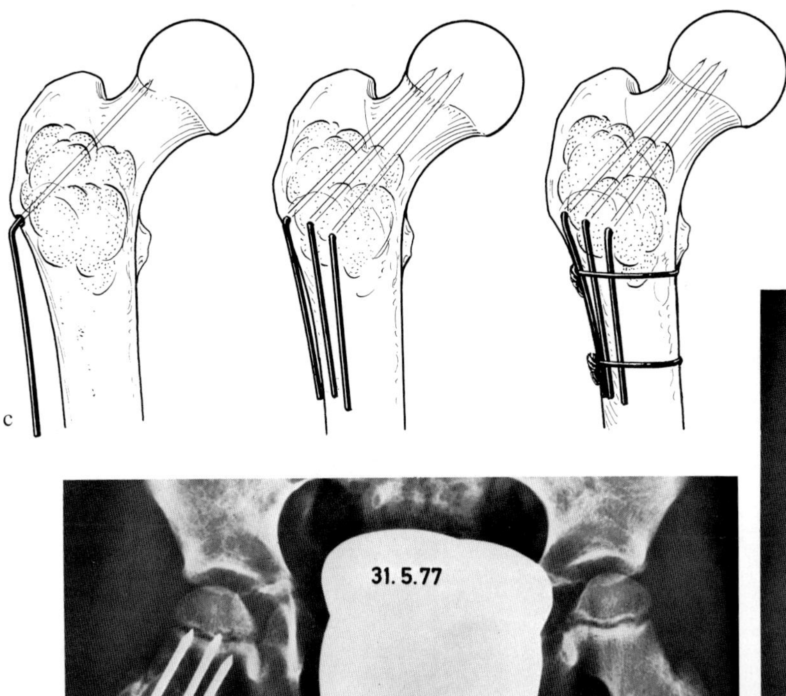

c

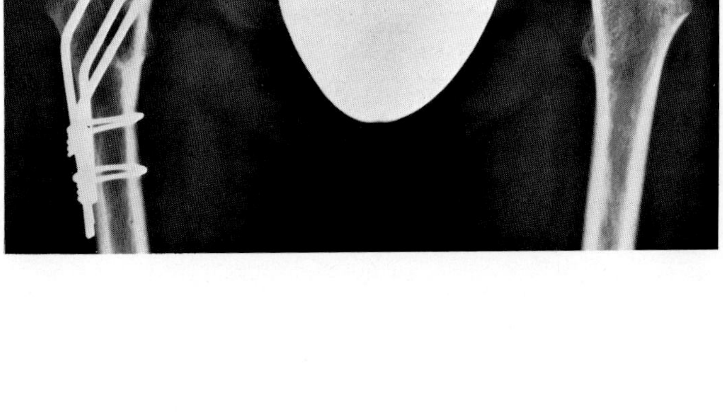

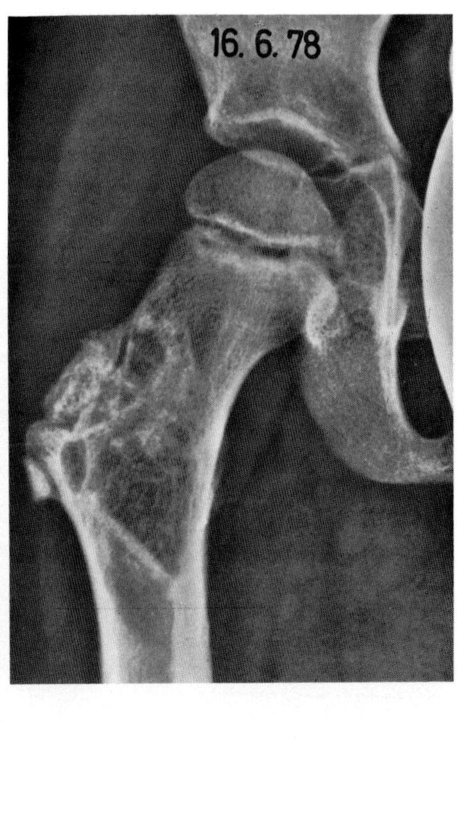

d, e

5.3 Combination of Kirschner Wire, Wire Loop, and External Fixator

The internal fixation techniques using Kirschner and cerclage wires are effective only if the bone fragments involved are resistant to compression. If they are not, as in the following example of a tumor, the two fragments must be held a normal distance apart by the external fixator, and the defect filled with autologous bone.

Example 1: Aneurysmal bone cyst of the intertrochanteric area with associated fracture in a child (Fig. 56)

The problem: The fracture and defect must heal without angular deformity or shortening of the limb.

The solution: After open reduction, two Schanz screws are inserted and stabilized by two external compression rods in such a way that shortening is prevented, i.e., the external fixator acts as a distractor. To secure the position of the fragments, four Kirschner wires are drilled into the distal fragment from the greater trochanter. The defect is filled with autologous cancellous bone. Finally, wire loops are passed around the proximal protruding ends of the Kirschner wires and anchored distally through lateral drill holes to create a tension band effect. The tension band is mainly for providing the necessary stability for mobilization following removal of the Schanz screws at 5 weeks.

Fig. 56a–d. Combined internal fixation with wire tension band and external fixator in a pathologic pertrochanteric fracture in a child.
A.S., ♂, age 6, No. 173341.
a *Fracture:* Juvenile bone cyst in proximal metaphysis of femur, causing pathologic fracture.
b *Plan of operation:* Lack of medial buttressing is compensated by the distraction of the Schanz screws and external fixator; lateral tension resistance is provided by the wire loop (tension band). Internal splinting is ensured by the Kirschner wires.
c *Postoperative roentgenogram.*
d *Fourteen months after operation:* No signs of recurrence, fracture healed

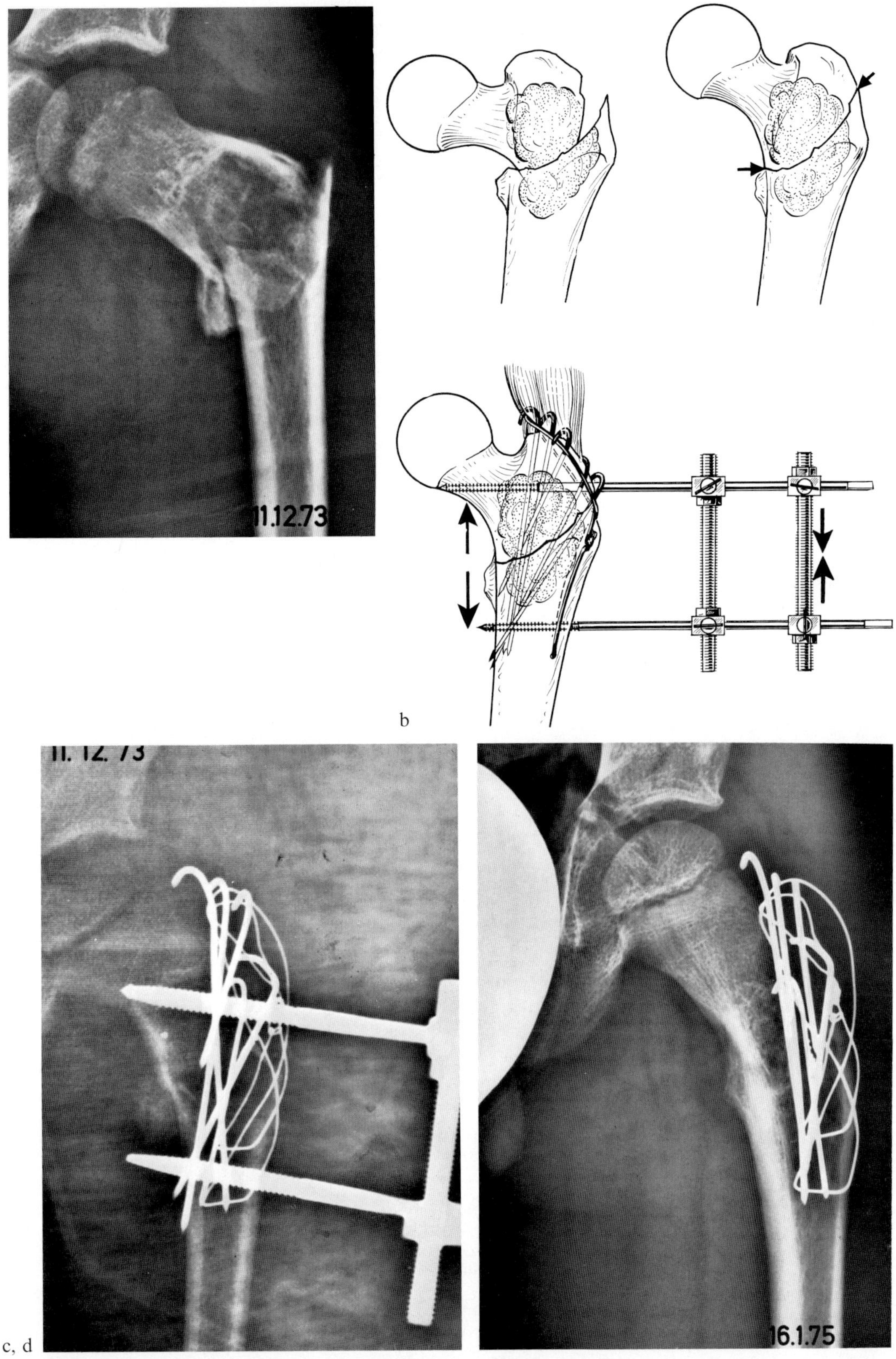

a

b

c, d

5.4 Tension Band Wires in Unusual Sites

Tension band wires can often provide a solution in cases where very small or very porotic bone fragments must be stabilized, yet the use of screws is contraindicated. This type of internal fixation is especially useful in hand surgery.

a–c

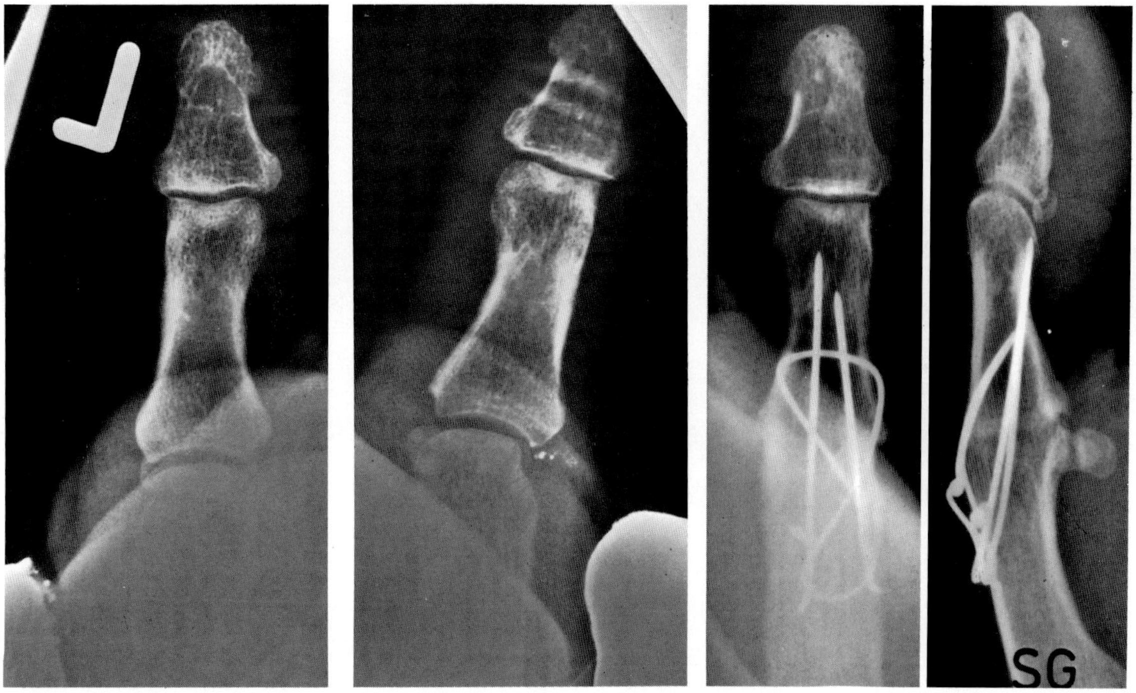

Fig. 57a–c. Tension band wiring for arthrodesis of the thumb in osteoporosis.
B.G., ♂, age 57, No. 180480.
a Unstable, painful basal thumb joint following rupture of collateral ulnar ligament.
b Stress roentgenogram.
c Healed arthrodesis

Example 1: Arthrodesis of the thumb (Fig. 57)

The problem: With chronic instability there is always some degree of osteoporosis, and the two phalanges are quite small.

The solution: The two near-parallel Kirschner wires determine the position of the arthrodesis, while the wire loop absorbs tension forces and provides interfragmental compression.

Example 2: Arthrodesis of the wrist in chronic polyarthritis (Fig. 58)

The problem: Screws and plates are of no use in the osteoporotic bone.

The solution: The arthrodesis is bridged by two thick Kirschner wires inserted from the carpus. A wire is looped around the free ends of the wires and drawn taut against the shaft of the radius, thus creating a tension band which, together with the wrist flexors, produces stabilizing axial compression in the arthrodesis.

Fig. 58 a–c. Tension band wiring for arthrodesis of the wrist in the presence of massive osteoporosis.
M.M., ♀, age 65, No. 146892.
a Severe, chronic, generalized polyarthritis; unstable, very painful wrists.
b *Operation:* Arthrodesis of the wrist with interposition of a bone graft. The thick Kirschner wires function as a splint and, together with the dorsal tension band wire applied under tension, form a stable internal fixation system.
c *One year after operation:* Good consolidation of arthrodesis

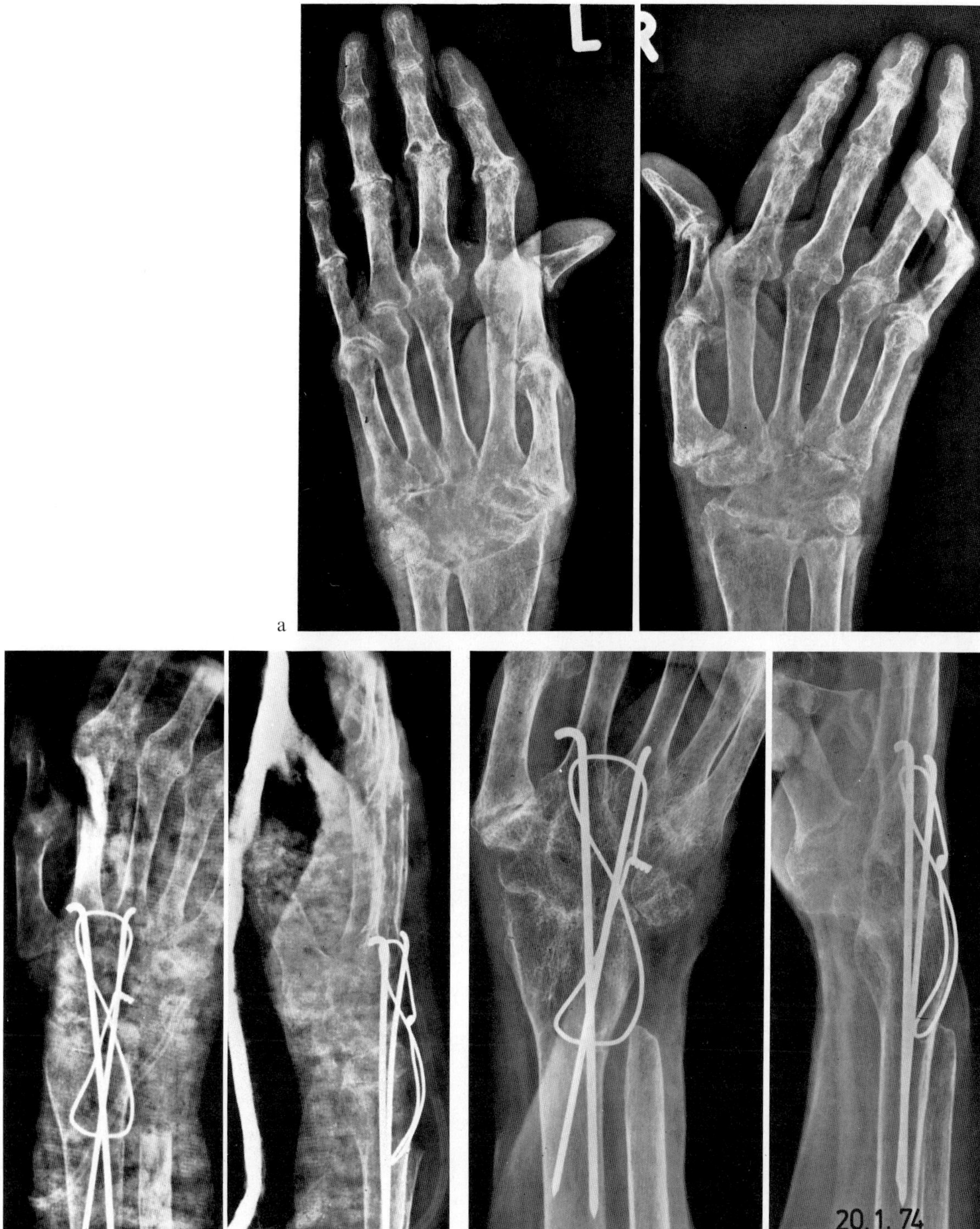

a

b

c

6 Anti-glide Plate

An internal fixation plate may fall into one of several categories, depending on its function (*Manual of Internal Fixation,* MÜLLER et al., 1977):

1. Static compression plate
2. Dynamic compression plate
3. Neutralization plate
4. Buttress plate.

In addition to these are two other types which perform specialized functions:

5. Bridge plate (e.g., for lengthening osteotomies, bone defects)
6. Anti-glide plate.

The purpose of the anti-glide plate is to prevent the fragments in an oblique fracture, osteotomy or pseudarthrosis from gliding upon each other when axial compressive forces are applied (Fig. 59). The axial compression may be produced by physiologic loads, the glide plate itself, a lag screw applied outside the glide plate, a second plate, or an external fixator.

Fig. 59. Principle of the anti-glide plate. A plate is fixed to the bone in such a way that it prevents the distal fragment from overriding when force is applied along the long axis of the bone. The distal fragment is firmly wedged between the plate and the fracture surface of the proximal fragment

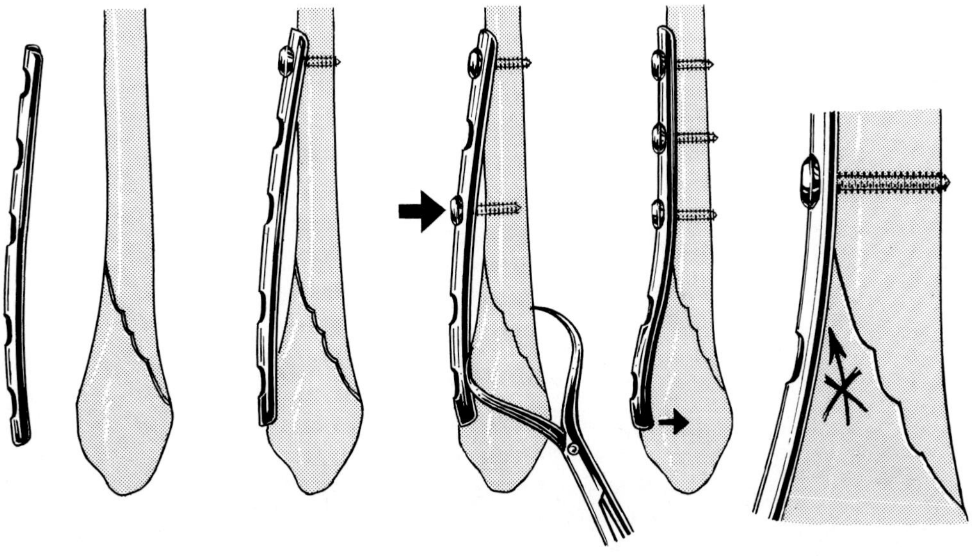

6.1 Anti-glide Plate and Stabilizing Compressive Loading

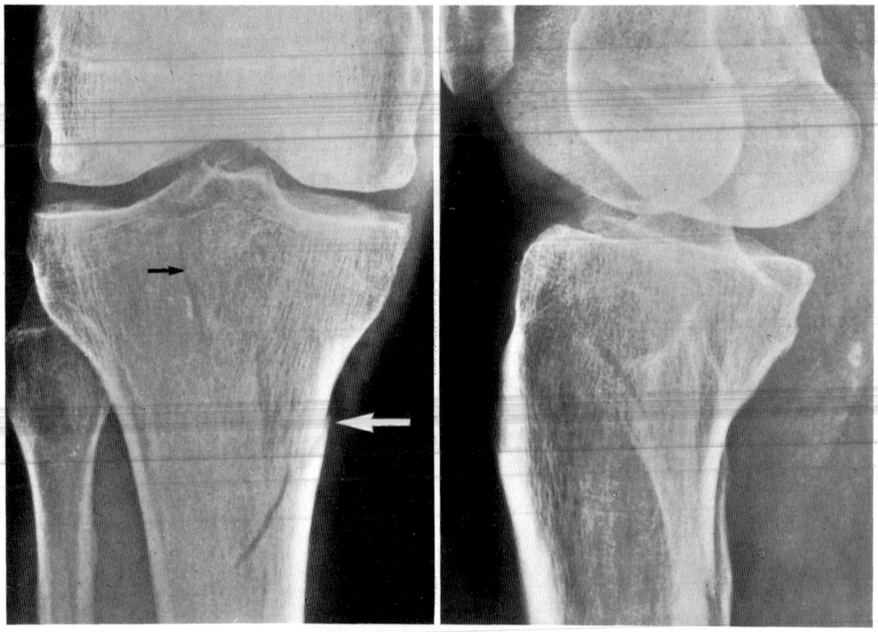

a

Example 1: Fracture of the tibial plateau: "one-hole anti-glide plate" (Fig. 60)

Even in simple split fractures, but especially in depressed and comminuted fractures, buttressing with a plate is indicated. The one-hole plate may offer the only possible means of buttressing the fracture or may be useful as a supplement to a buttress plate.

The problem: Gliding of the fragments must be reliably prevented with a minimum implantation of foreign material (here: without a plate).

The solution: The spike formed by the tibial border is kept from gliding by pressing it against the main distal fragment with the aid of a contoured washer. The drill hole for the one-hole plate must be cut directly through the fracture line (the only instance where this is permitted in internal fixation).

Fig. 60a–d. One-hole anti-glide plate. C.R., ♂, age 34, No. 196498.
a Split fracture of the tibial plateau.
b *Operation:* Transverse lag-screw fixation.
c *Prevention of fragment gliding:* The washer of the distal screw presses the tip of the distal fragment against the main fragment. This requires that the screw be inserted through the fracture line (the only exception to the rule).
d *Two years after injury:* Complete recovery

b
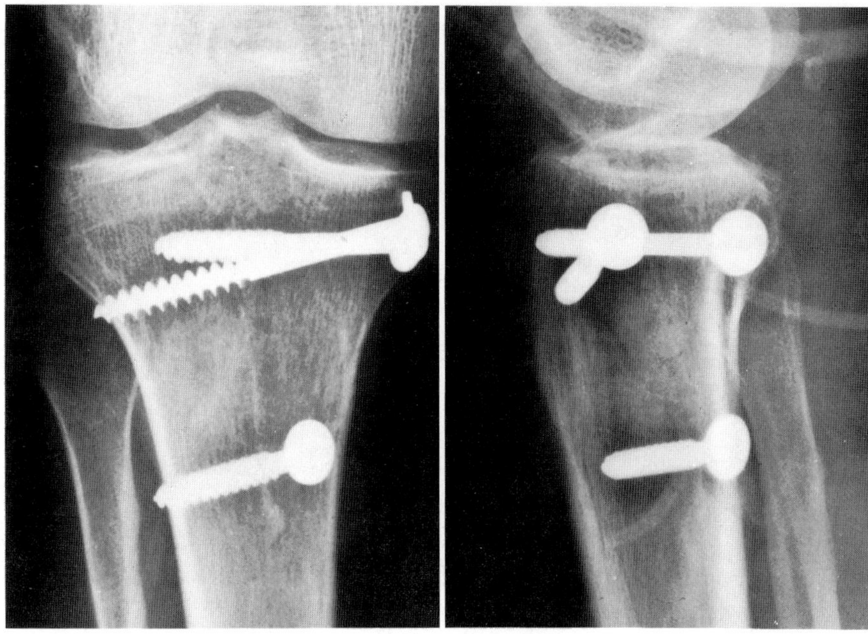

c
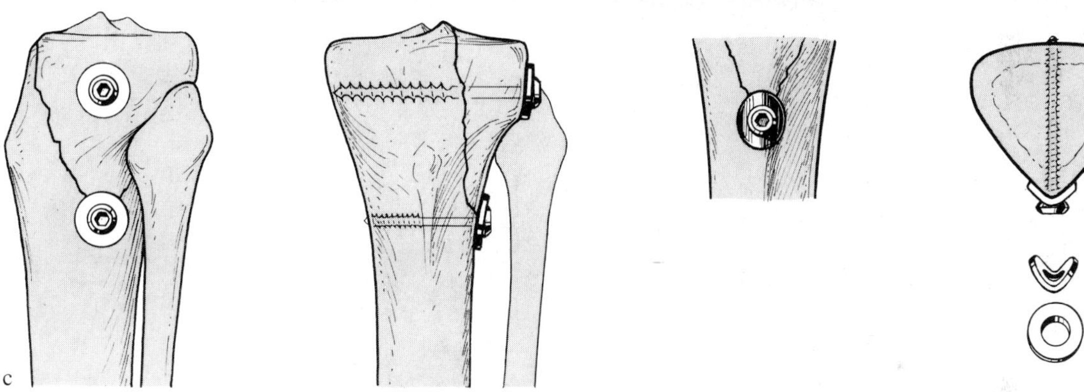

d
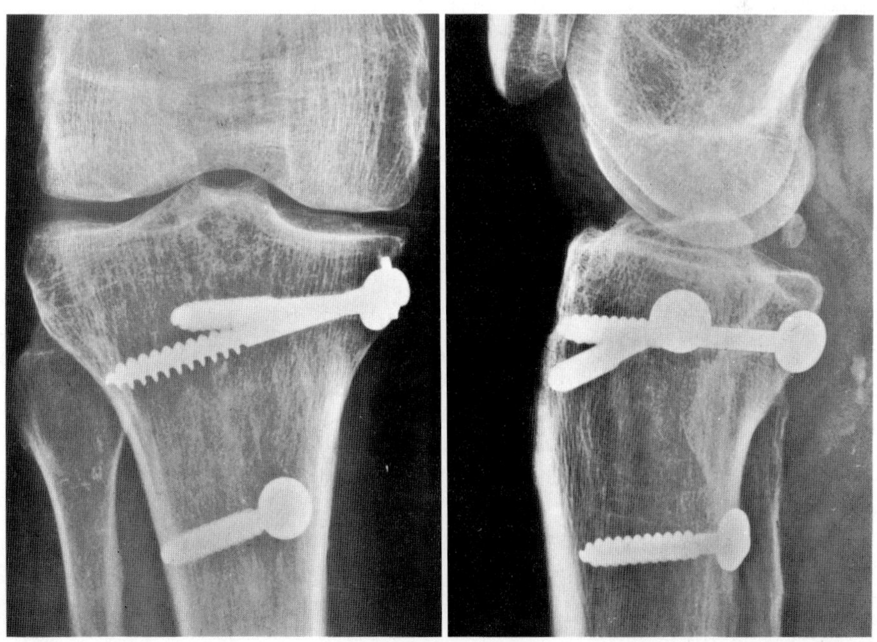

Example 2: Fracture of the head of the radius: two-hole anti-glide plate (Fig. 61)

The problem: Direct screw fixation is sometimes impossible because the fragments are too small or have further comminution.

The solution: After digital reduction of the "chisel" fragments, the fragments are redisplaced either by direct screw insertion or with the aid of a small, contoured, two-hole anti-glide plate. Due to the small size of the fragment to be buttressed, screw fixation through the plate is not possible, but neither is it essential; the fragment is held in place by the end of the plate.

Fig. 61 a–c. Small anti-glide plate in a radial head fracture.
S.V., ♀, age 42, No. 209552.
a Depressed fracture of radial head plateau, small chisel fragment.
b *Operation:* Transverse lag-screw fixation, screw heads countersunk below cartilage surface. The comminuted zone is compressed and kept from gliding by the small two-hole plate.
c *Four months after injury:* Fracture healed without complications

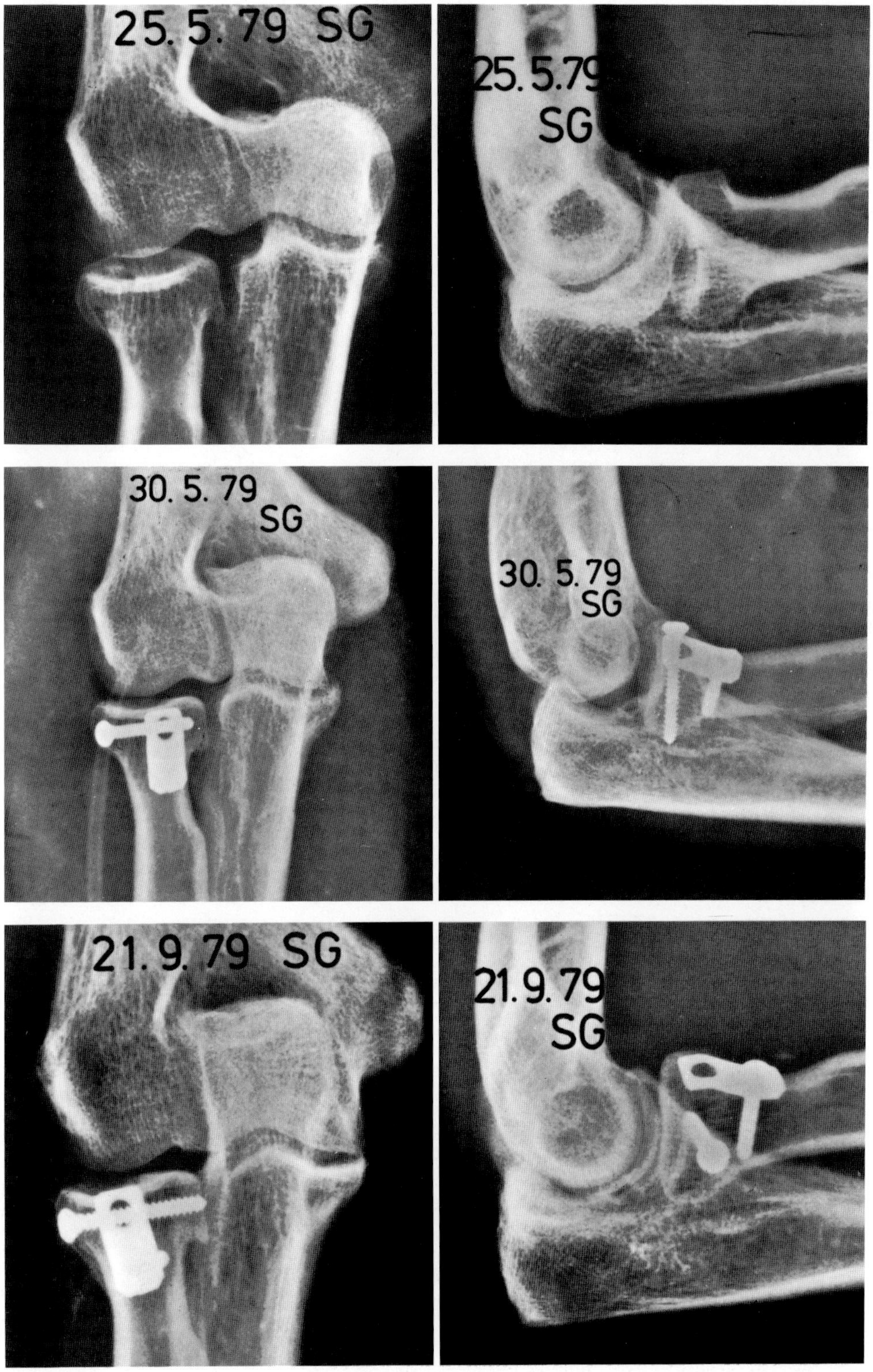

a

b

c

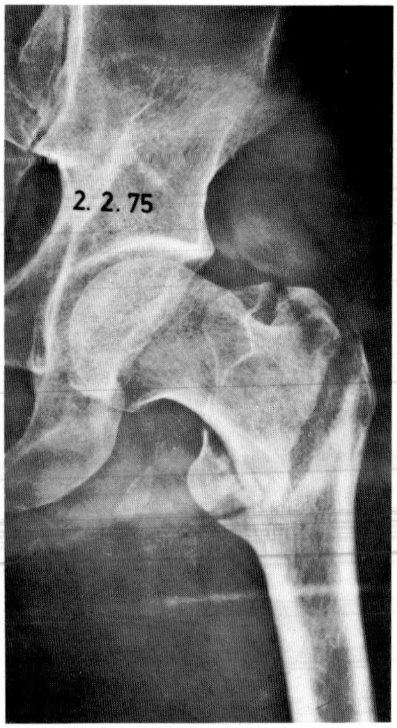

a

Example 3: Pertrochanteric fracture of the femur with marked gliding tendency: multiple-hole anti-glide plate (Fig. 62)

In younger patients with a pertrochanteric fracture, the goal is fracture healing with complete anatomic restoration, without shortening, varus, valgus, or rotational deformity.

The problem: The proximal fragment has a stubborn tendency to glide medialward down the inclined fracture plane relative to the distal fragment. None of the standard internal fixation techniques can prevent this with certainty.

The solution: Prior to reduction, a contoured three- or four-hole semitubular plate is mounted on the calcar in the medullary cavity of the proximal fragment. When the fracture is reduced, the free end of the plate enters the medullary cavity of the distal fragment. Now the proximal fragment can no longer glide, i.e., the fracture has a firm medial buttress and can be anatomically reduced and fixed. A screw can be inserted in the empty caudal plate hole through an opening in the fracture line.

Fig. 62a–e. Anti-glide plate in a pertrochanteric fracture.
W.W., ♂, age 32, No. 184479.
a Pertrochanteric fracture.
b *Problem encountered at operation and its solution:* The cortices cannot be stably aligned on the medial side. In the same way that the wheel rim keeps the train on the track, the anti-glide plate can keep the fragments aligned: The small plate screwed to the calcar in the medullary cavity prevents "derailing" of the proximal fragment.
c *Operation:* Anti-glide plate, tension banding and splinting.
d *Four months after injury:* Fracture healing without deformity.
e *Two years after injury, after removal of implants:* The small intramedullary plate must be left in place; recovery is complete in other respects

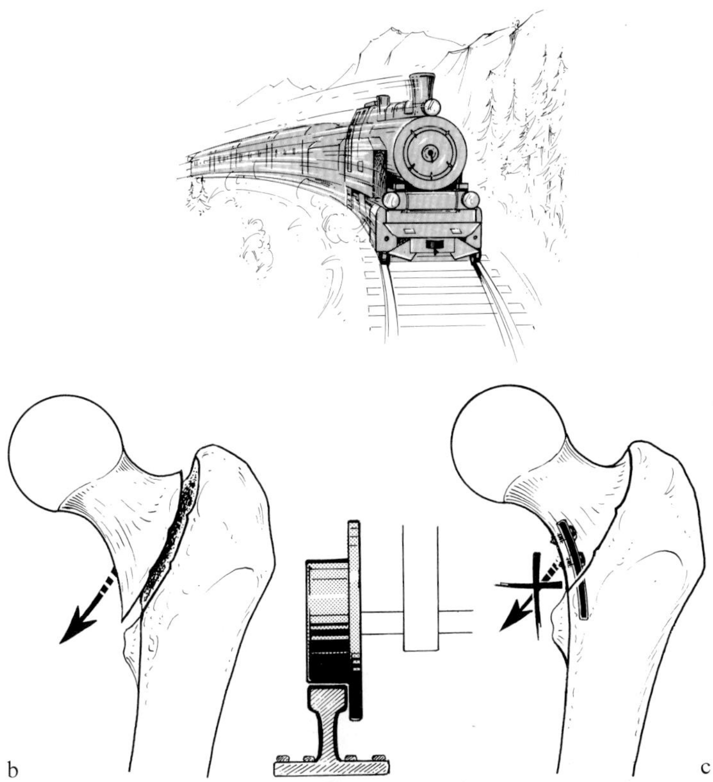

b

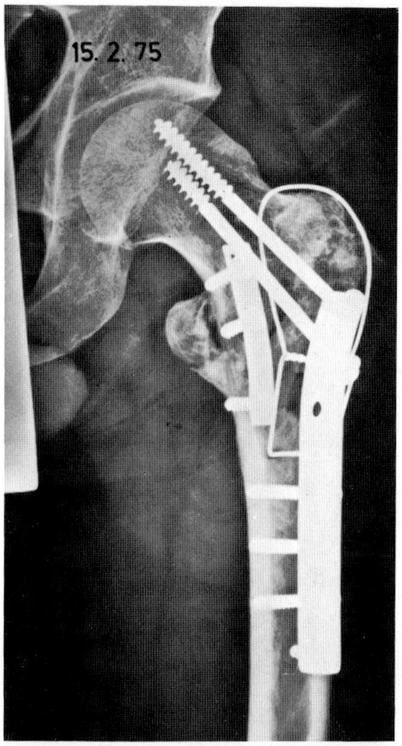

c

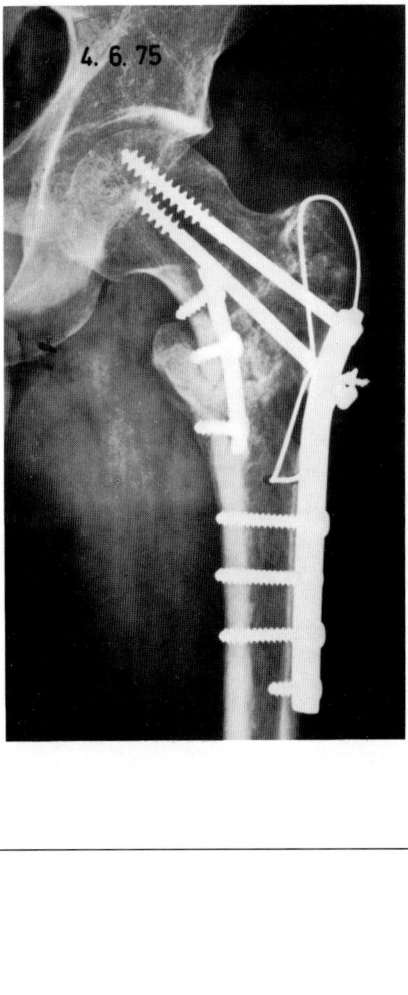

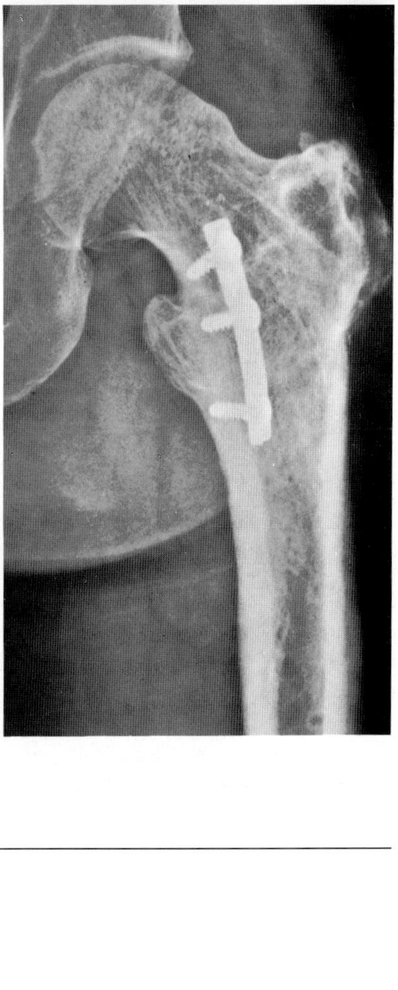

d, e

6.2 Anti-glide Plate with Supplementary Compression

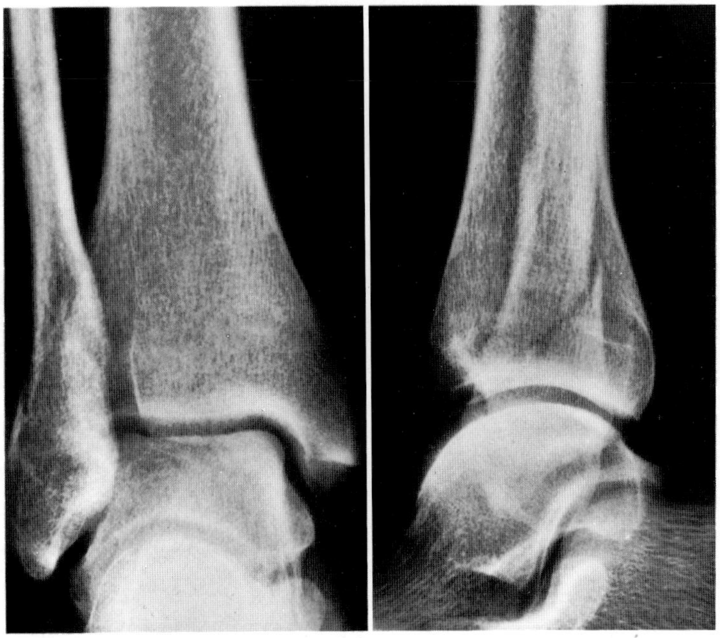

a

Fig. 63a–c. Small posterior plate and malleolar screw.
R.R., ♂, age 58, No. 189525.
a Type-B fracture-dislocation.
b *Internal fixation:* Small posterior anti-glide plate. Additional compression obtained with doubly oblique malleolar lag screw.
c *Six months after injury:* Complete recovery

Example 1: Type-B oblique fracture of the distal fibula: anti-glide plate with doubly oblique malleolar lag screw (Fig. 63)

The problem: Axial compression would be desirable to improve stability after reduction of the fracture, but this is very difficult to achieve by means of conventional operative techniques, even lateral plating.

The solution: A one-third tubular plate is applied to the posterior or posterolateral side of the distal fibula, thereby pressing the tip of the distal fragment securely against the proximal fragment (Fig. 64). Stabilizing interfragmental compression is provided by a separate lag screw.

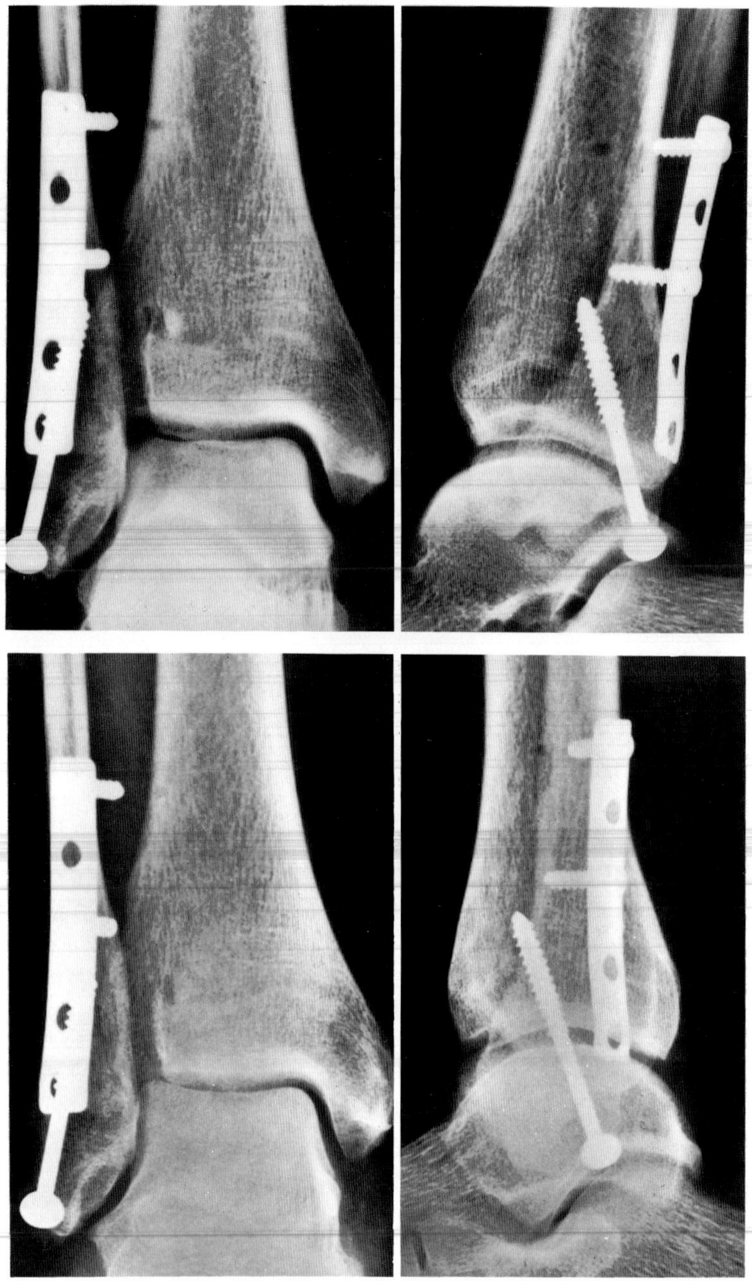

b

c

Fig. 63b, c. Legend see p. 123

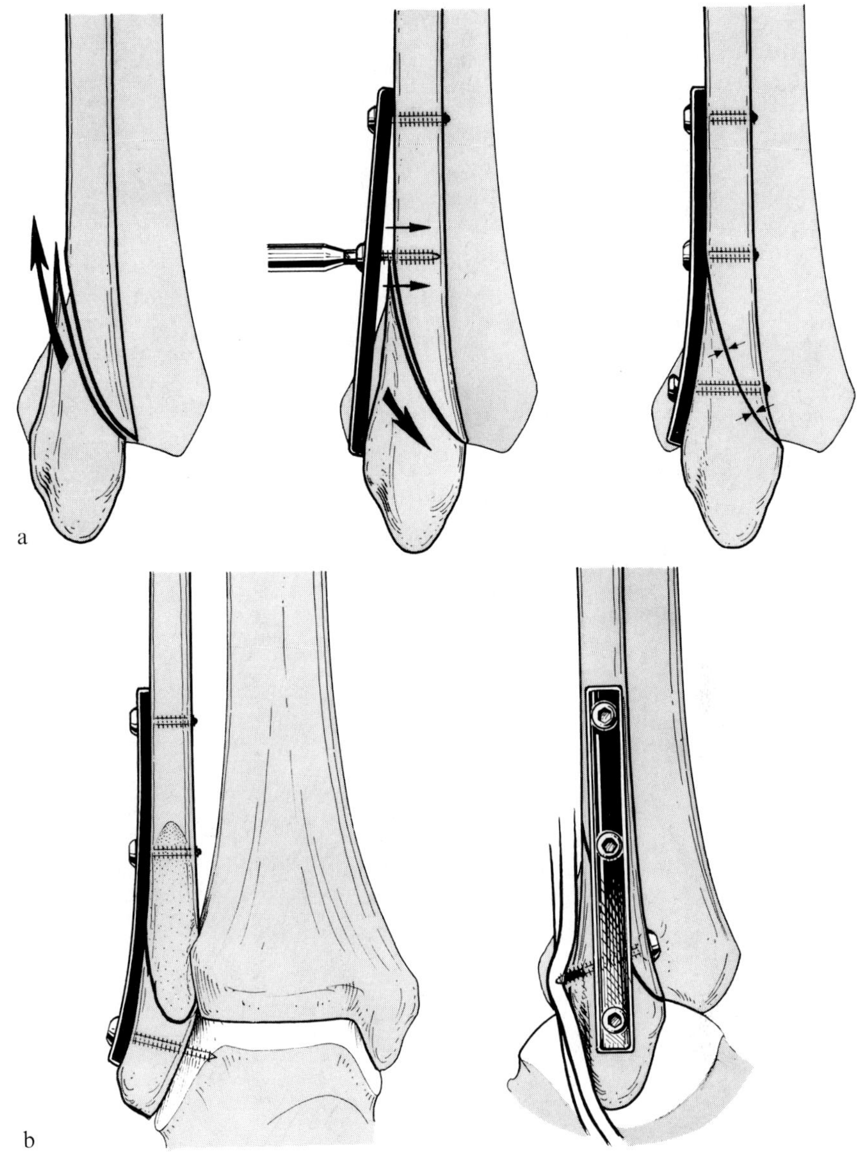

Fig. 64a, b. Anti-glide plate with supplemental interfragmental compression. **a** *Anti-glide plate in type-B fracture of the ankle joint:* The one-third tubular plate applied to the posterior surface of the fibula is attached first proximally, then distally. The plate prevents proximal gliding of the distal fragment. In some cases a lag screw may be inserted through the plate to provide supplementary interfragmental compression. **b** *The hazards of lateral plating in type-B fractures of the ankle joint:* The distal screw can easily penetrate the ankle joint. An overlong lag screw inserted in the AP direction can damage the peroneus tendons a 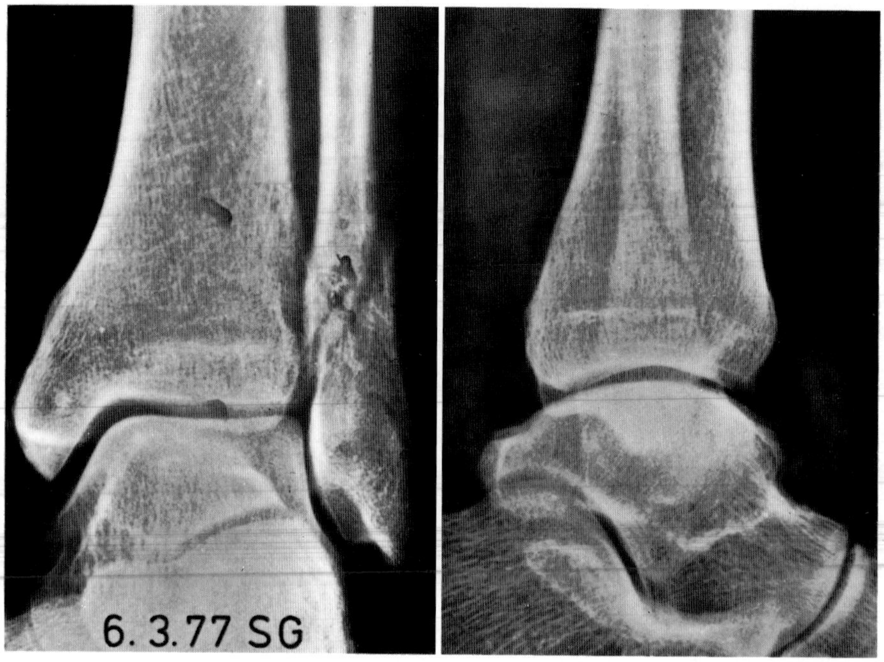

Example 2: Type-B distal fibular fracture: anti-glide plate with lag screw inserted through the plate (Fig. 65)

The problem: Various biomechanical configurations can arise once the anti-glide plate is applied. The course of the oblique spiral fracture may be such that a lag screw inserted outside the plate would tend to disturb the reduction.

The solution: The lag screw is inserted posteroanteriorly through the distal hole of the anti-glide plate, preferably gaining purchase in the anterior tubercle of the fibula. Its main purpose is to exert stabilizing interfragmental, rather than axial, compression.

Fig. 65a–c. Anti-glide plate with through-the-plate lag screw in a type-B fracture of the fibula.
S. A., ♀, age 60, No. 205934.
a Type-B fracture-dislocation.
b *Internal fixation:* The small posterior plate is supplemented by a lag screw inserted across the fracture line.
c *Six months after injury:* Complete recovery

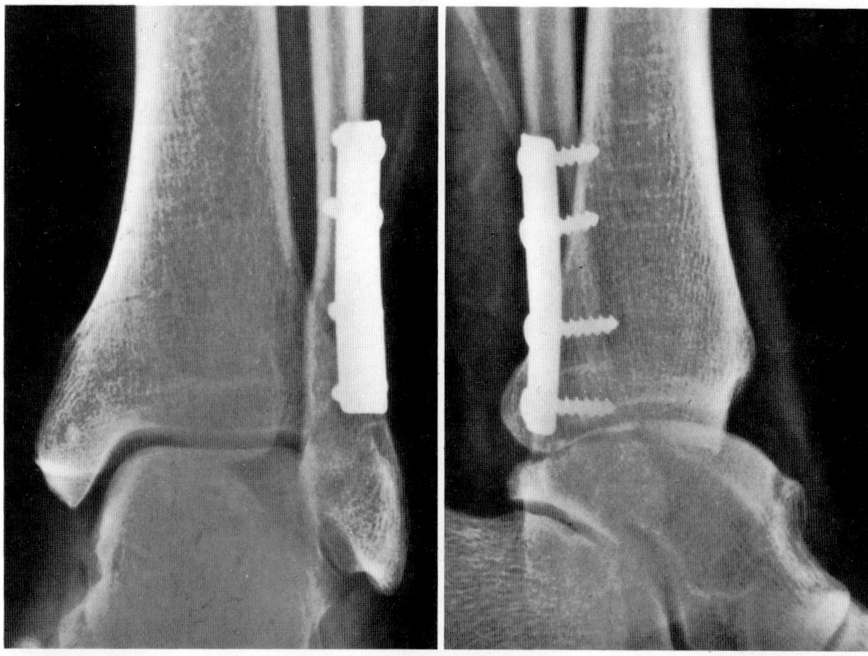

b

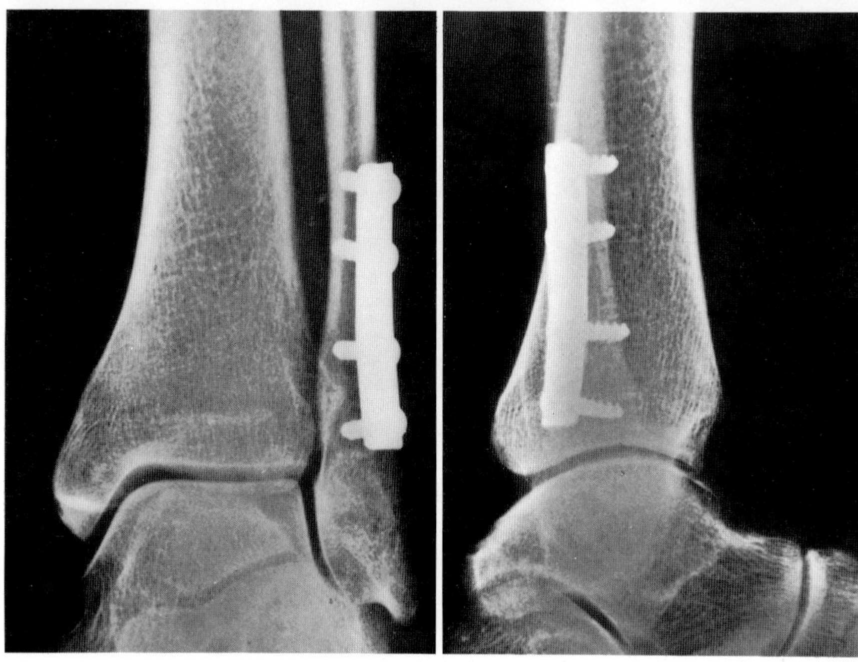

c

Example 3: Comminuted supracondylar fracture of the humerus: anti-glide plate with interfragmental lag screws (Fig. 66)

The problem: The fracture has disrupted the medial buttress of the distal humerus, which must be restored.

The solution: A semitubular plate is screwed from the main medial fragment to the torsion "butterfly" component, its distal end encompassing the crest of the medial buttress. Two lag screws above and below the olecranon fossa produce interfragmental compression.

Fig. 66a–c. Anti-glide plate in a distal humeral fracture with an interrupted medial pillar.
M.L., ♀, age 61, No. 114719.
a Comminuted fracture.
b *Operation:* Screw fixation alone does not adequately stabilize the medial pillar. The anti-glide plate solves this problem by simple means.
c *Ten months after injury:* Uneventful fracture union, normal elbow mobility

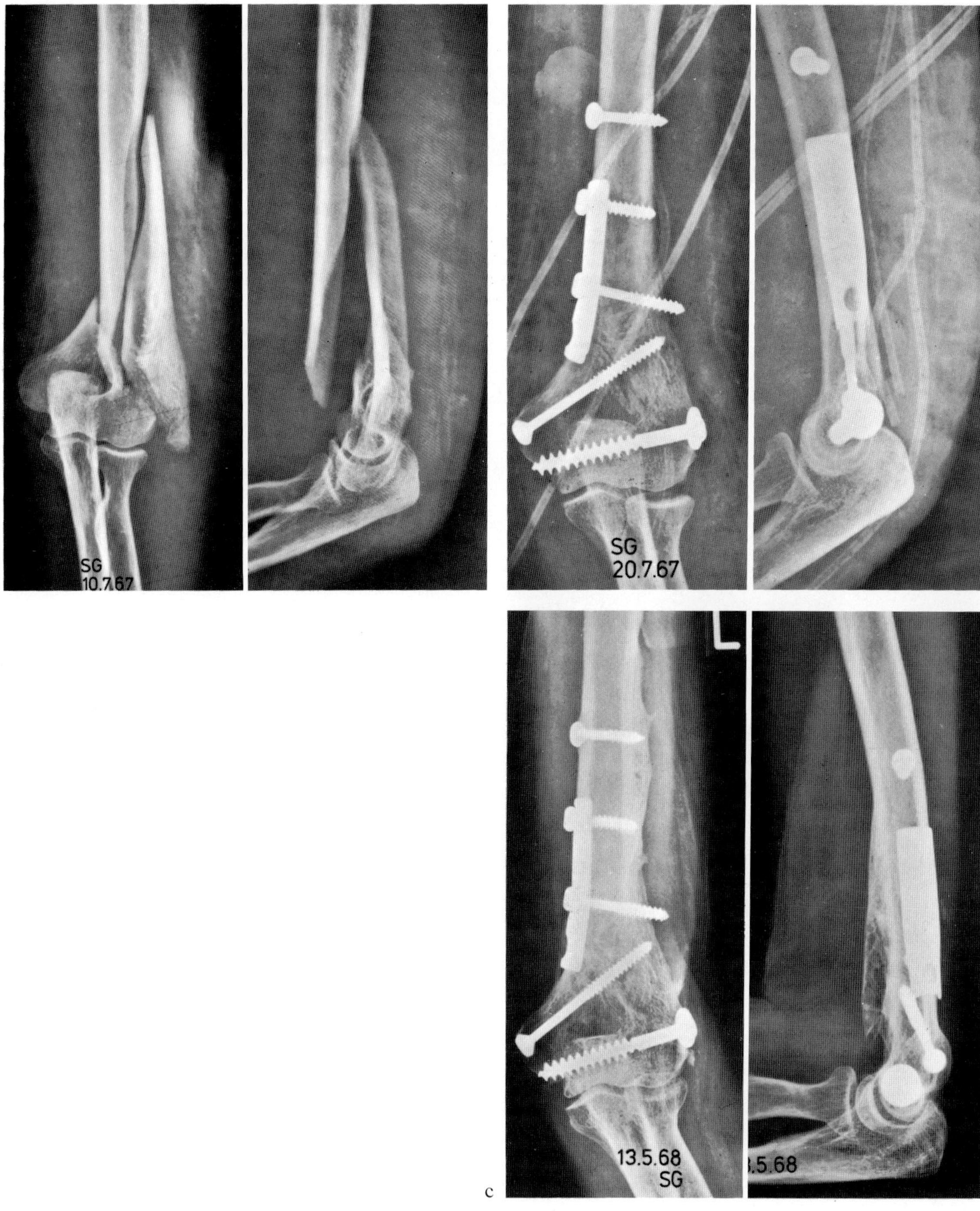

a, b

c

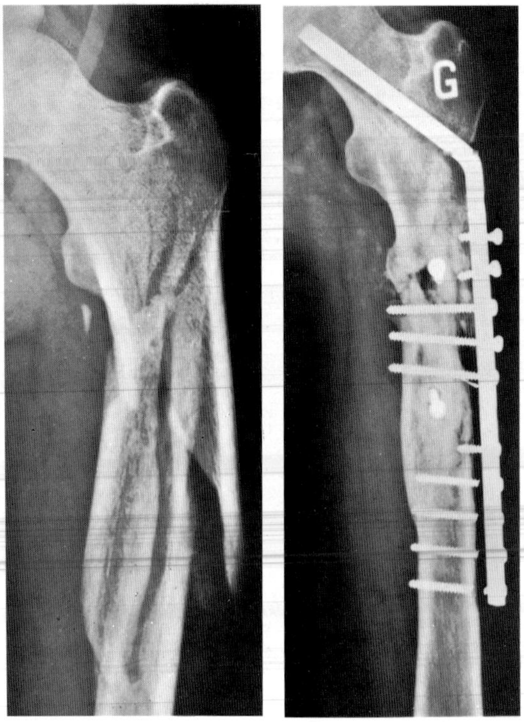

a, b

Example 4: Oblique pseudarthrosis of the femur: anti-glide plate combined with tension band plate (Fig. 67)

The problem: The pseudarthrosis is best repaired by compressive internal fixation combined with tension banding. A condylar plate alone cannot perform this function, because the pseudarthrosis lies on the frontal plane. Gliding of the fragments could be prevented by interfragmental lag screws inserted perpendicular to the tension band plate, but the shaft is too osteoporotic to anchor the screws securely.

The solution: A narrow five-hole plate is mounted on the anterior side of the femur with three screws through the distal fragment, so that the tip of the proximal fragment is pressed against the main distal fragment. Then a tension band plate is attached to the lateral surface, allowing very strong stabilizing, axial compression to be exerted without causing fragmental overriding and consequent shortening of the bone. Finally, lag screws are driven into the free holes of the anti-glide plate to create additional interfragmental compression.

Fig. 67 a–f. Anti-glide plate in oblique pseudarthrosis of the femoral shaft. E.R., ♂, age 24, No. 136787.
a Subtrochanteric comminuted fracture.
b *Nine months after injury:* Infected pseudarthrosis.
c *Two and a half years after injury:* Infected femoral pseudarthrosis coursing in AP-oblique direction.
d *Pseudarthrosis surgery:* First the anti-glide plate is applied to the anterior side to give the pseudarthrosis compressive strength. The lateral plate functions as a tension band in the usual fashion, since the anterior plate prevents gliding of the fragments.
e *Eleven months after operation:* Pseudarthrosis healed, implants removed.
f *Two years after operation:* Pseudarthrosis and infection are healed

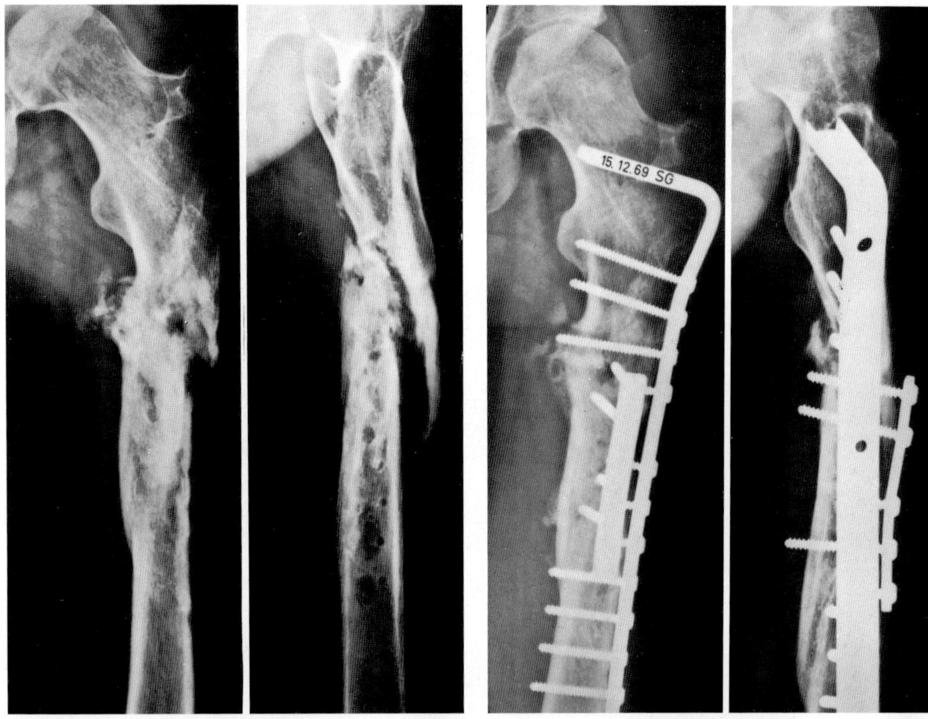

c, d

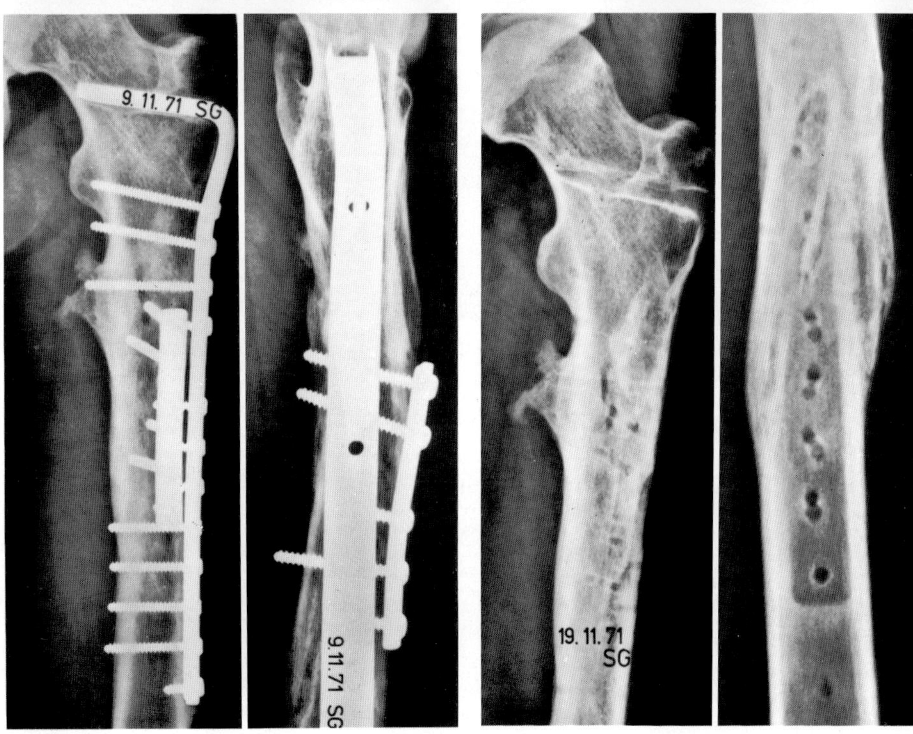

e, f

Example 5: Anti-glide plate combined with an external fixator (Fig. 68)

The problem: The external fixator represents a great advance in the management of third-degree open tibial fractures from the standpoint of promoting soft-tissue healing. It does little to promote healing of the fracture itself, and secondary operations are therefore usually necessary for this purpose. It would be desirable for the external fixator to play a more direct role in the promotion of fracture union.

The solution: We have found that in open fractures managed primarily with external fixation, a highly accurate primary reduction is important in terms of bone healing. But minimal internal fixation can be applied only in areas where the implant will be adequately covered by viable soft tissue. "Minimal" fixation in this case includes such procedures as sparing screw fixation of the tibial fragments, plate fixation of the fibula (auxiliary internal fixation), and the placement of an anti-glide plate. With the latter, the blood supply to the fragment tip is less compromised than in the case of screw fixation.

Fig. 68a–c. External fixator supplemented by minimal internal fixation. In the tibia, it is desirable in terms of soft tissue healing and anterior tibial muscle function to mount the external fixator as a compressor on the medial tibial surface. For this a certain axial compressive stability is necessary. This is present in a transverse fracture, but must be created in oblique fractures. There are three possible means of achieving this:
a Lag screw across the oblique fracture.
b Plate fixation of the fibula in the transverse or short oblique tibial fracture for augmentation of the patient's ability.
c *Anti-glide plate.* It prevents the fragments in an oblique fracture from gliding upon each other while causing minimal interference with the blood supply to the fragment tip

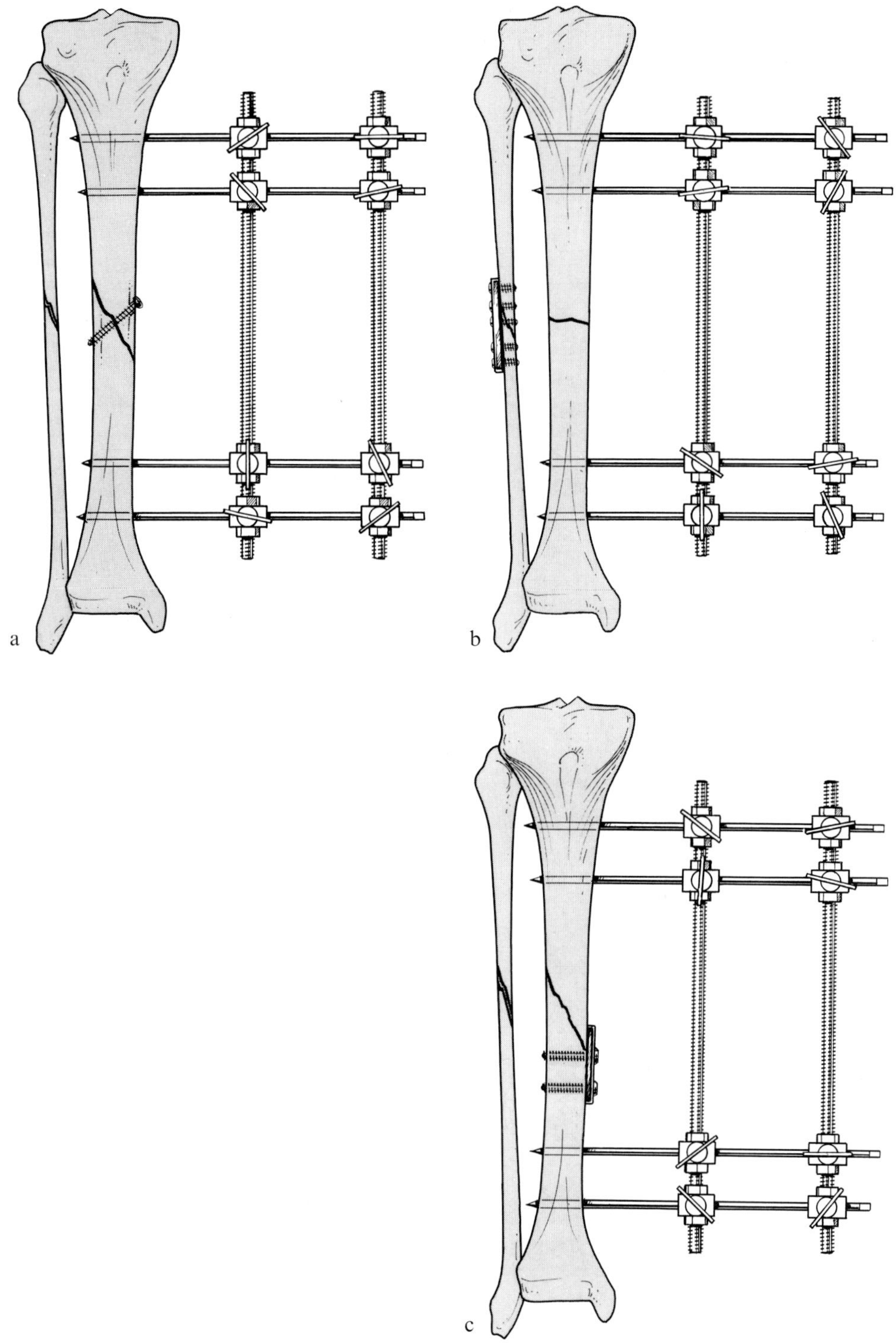
a
b
c

7 Plating of the Vertebral Column

Primary, secondary, temporary, or permanent spinal fusions may be employed for the stabilization of unstable vertebral fractures. Plating is indicated if it offers the most straightforward means of achieving the therapeutic goal. Sometimes the goal can be reached only by the simultaneous application of anterior and posterior measures or by successive interbody fusion and fixation/bone grafting from a posterior approach (or vice versa).

The following partial measures may be necessary:

The open reduction of dislocations with facet locking
The removal of fragments impinging on the dural sac from the vertebral adnexa
The stabilization of unstable vertebral adnexa
Temporary or permanent posterior fusion.

Of the many procedures that may be carried out on the vertebral column from a posterior approach, three unusual measures are described below.

7.1 Hook Plate

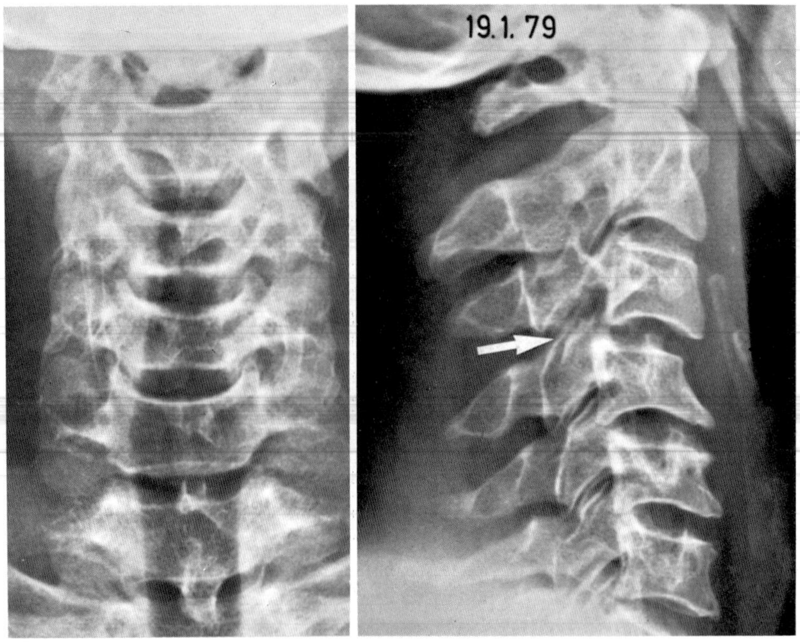

a

Example 1: Fracture-dislocation of the cervical spine with facet locking and fracture of an articular process (Fig. 69)

The problem: Not every dislocation with facet locking is stable after reduction. As a result of ligamentous tears and especially the partial fracture of an articular process of the dislocated vertebra, reduction leaves a rotational instability which occasionally goes unrecognized until surgery. Thus, the injured segment is more stable before reduction than after.

The solution: A straight four-hole small-fragment plate is bent into the shape of a hook and screwed to the lateral surface of the dislocated vertebra with the hooked portion placed over the laminal ridge of the adjacent vertebra.

Fig. 69a–f. Small plate with "anchoring" function.
H.J., ♂, age 45, No. 225222.
a, b Dislocation of C-3–C-4.
c *Operation:* After open reduction, two small one-third tubular plates are bent so that the hooked portion fits around the C-4 lamina, while the plate screws gain purchase in the pedicle and body of C-3. Interspinous fusion with bone graft.
d The system gains its stability in a manner analogous to that of a ship riding at anchor.
e, f *Four months after injury:* Reduction stable, fusion solid

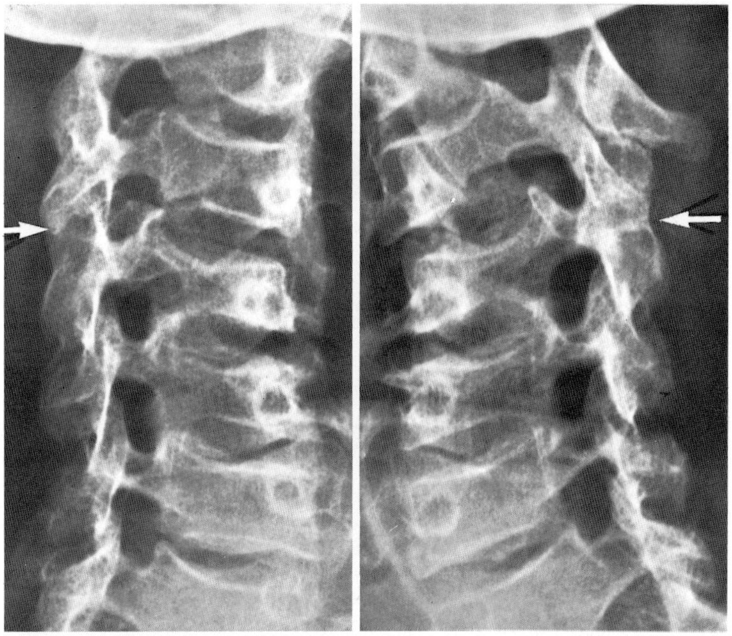

b

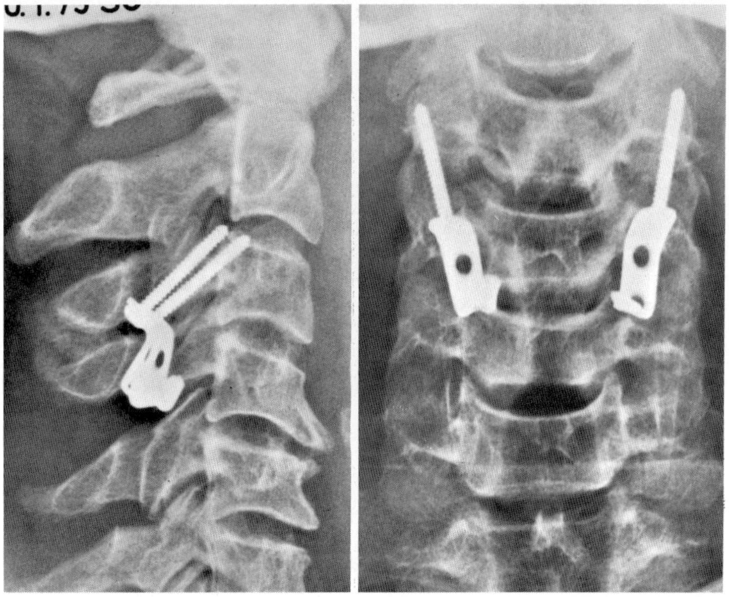

c

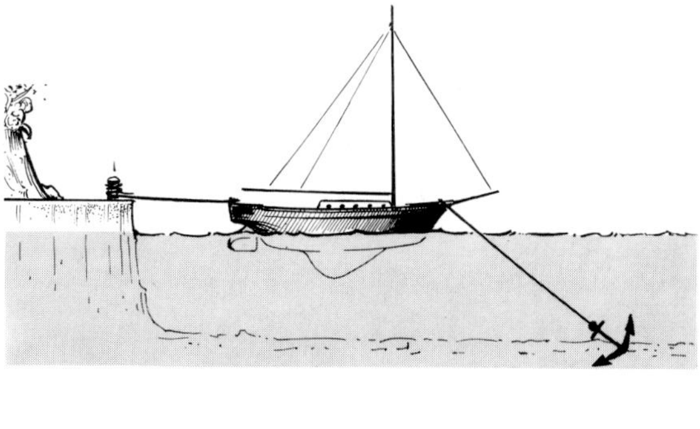

d

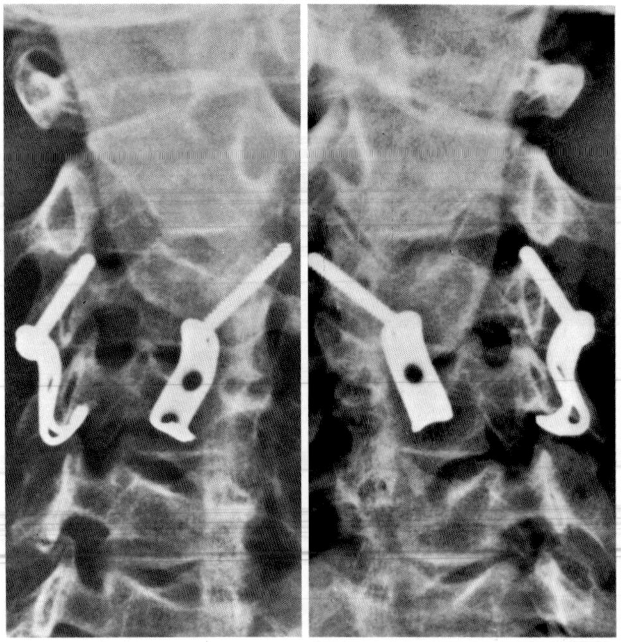

e

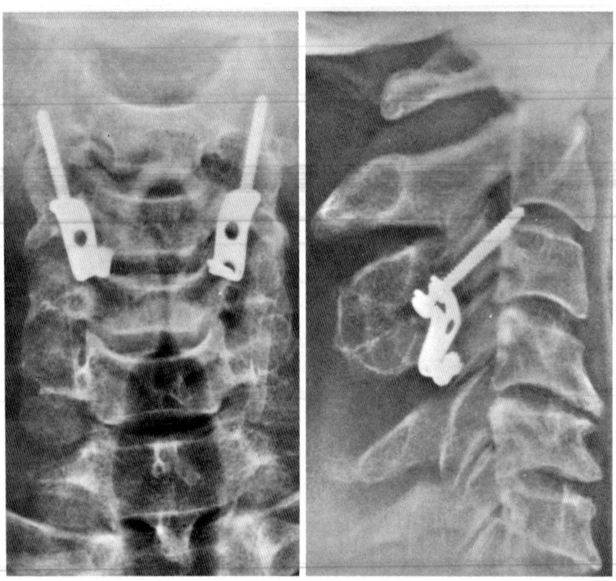

f

Fig. 69e, f. Legend see p. 136

7.2 "Articular Plate"

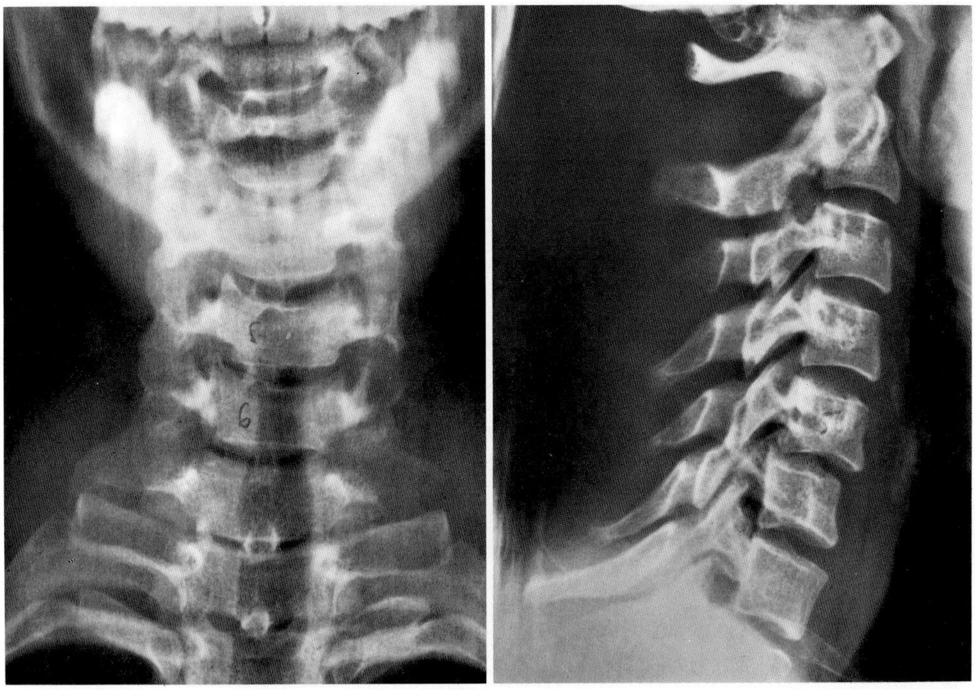

a

Fig. 70a–e. Two-hole plate as articular process in the cervical spine.
S.G., ♀, age 31, No. 223557.
a Fracture-dislocation of C-5–C-6, right-sided C-5 root paralysis.
b *Tomography:* The right-sided cranial articular process of C-6 is fractured, allowing the rotational subluxation of C-5. There is an associated partial fracture of the posterior lip of the vertebral body.
c *Operation:* After open reduction, the fractured process is replaced with a small two-hole plate, the caudal end of which is screwed tightly to the pedicle. This is supplemented by posterior fusion with an H-graft, reinforced with wire.
d *Six months after operation:* Fusion is solid.
e *One year after injury, after implant removal:* Patient free of complaints, no instability

Example 1: Dislocation of the cervical spine with fracture of an articular process of the adjacent vertebra (Fig. 70)

The problem: Rotational instability persists after reduction, because the fractured articular process of the adjacent vertebra offers no opposing surface for the caudal articular process of the dislocated vertebra. This situation first becomes evident at operation.

The solution: The fractured articular process is replaced by a small two-hole plate screwed to the base of the process. This creates a new bearing surface and restores rotational stability.

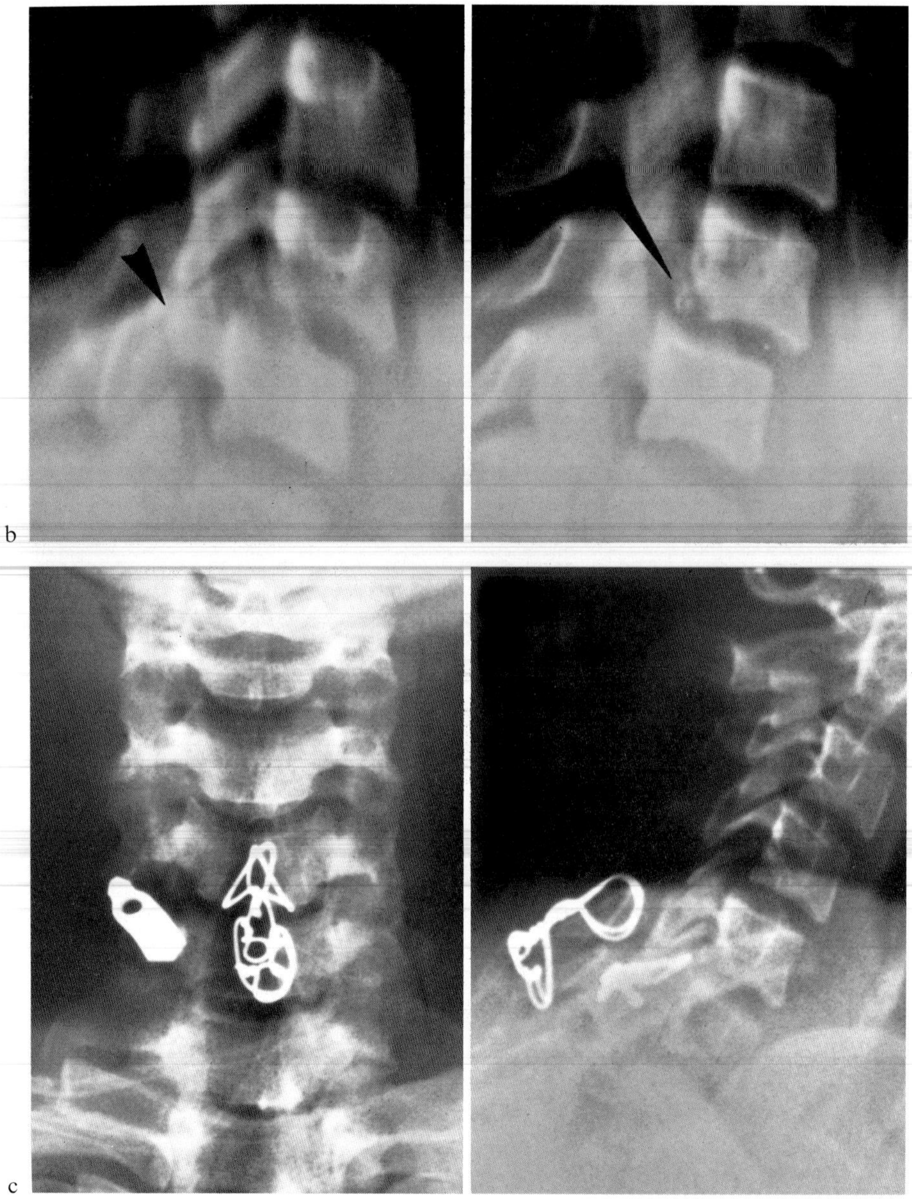

Fig. 70 b–e. Legend see p. 139

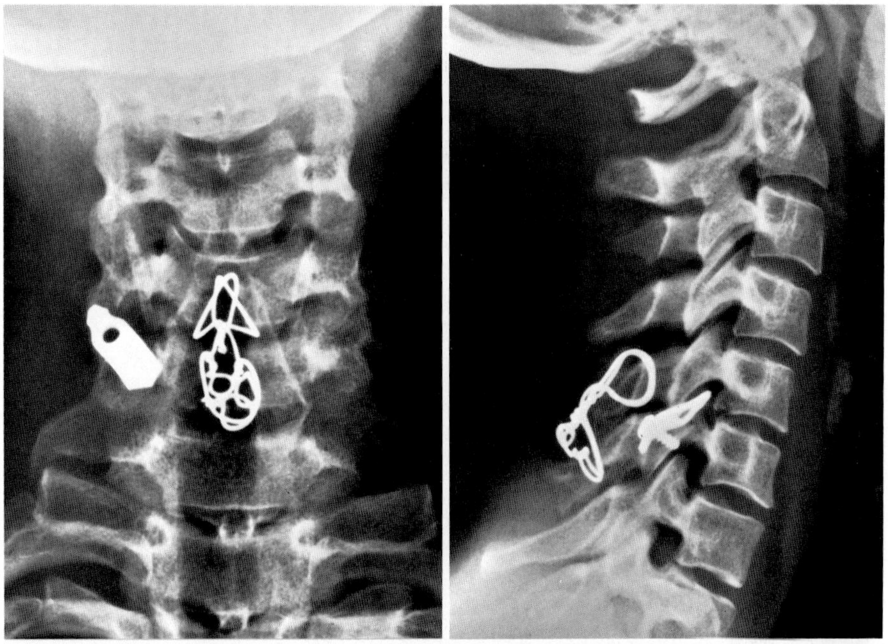

d

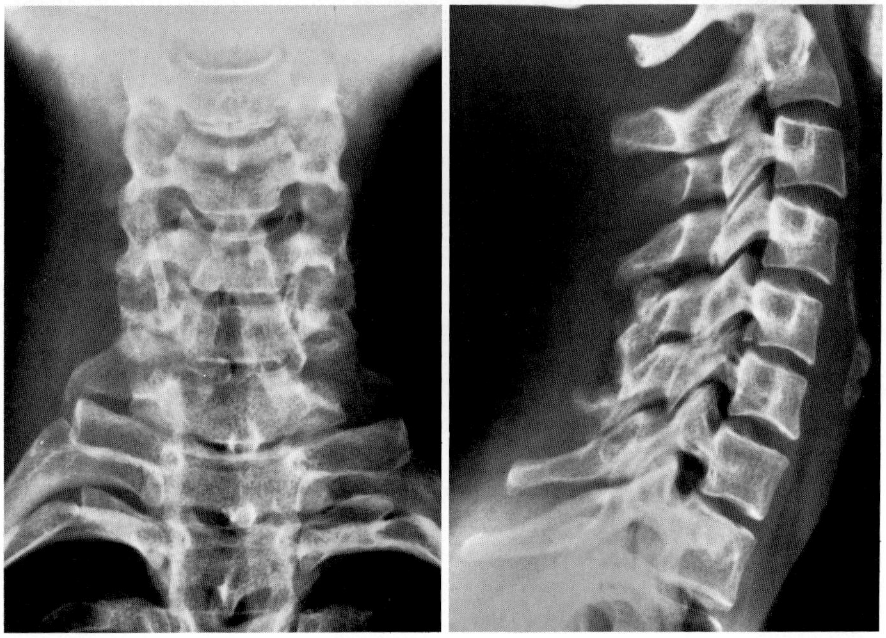

e

7.3 Posterior Plating (Roy-Camille, Zerah)

a 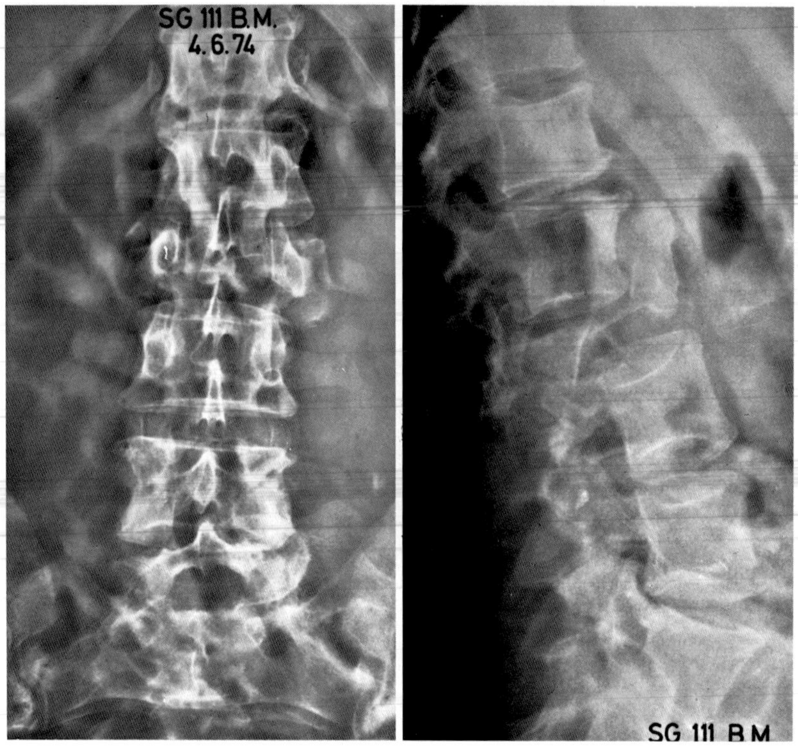

Example 1: Unstable fracture-dislocation of L-2–L-3 with incomplete paraplegia (Fig. 71)

The problem: After the operative removal of fragments impinging on the dural sac, requiring a laminectomy, the vertebral column is left with a high-grade instability. An internal fixation stable enough to withstand exercise is desirable to maintain decompression, facilitate nursing care, and promote rapid and anatomically favorable fracture union.

The solution: Plates of the correct length, contour, and hole spacing are attached laterally by screws inserted through the pedicles into the vertebral body. In the same operation, a posterior bone graft is placed and is supplemented if necessary by interbody fusion.

Fig. 71 a–c. Plating for an unstable fracture-dislocation of L-2–L-3 with progressing paraplegia.
B.M., ♀, age 62, No. 178036.
a Burst fracture of second lumbar vertebral body and dislocation of L-2–L-3.
b *Operation:* After inspection of the spinal canal, cord decompression, and reconstruction of the dura, the spine is stabilized with two posterior plates. The screws are driven through the pedicles into the vertebral bodies.
c *Three years and 9 months after injury:* Complete neurologic recovery, vertebral column stable

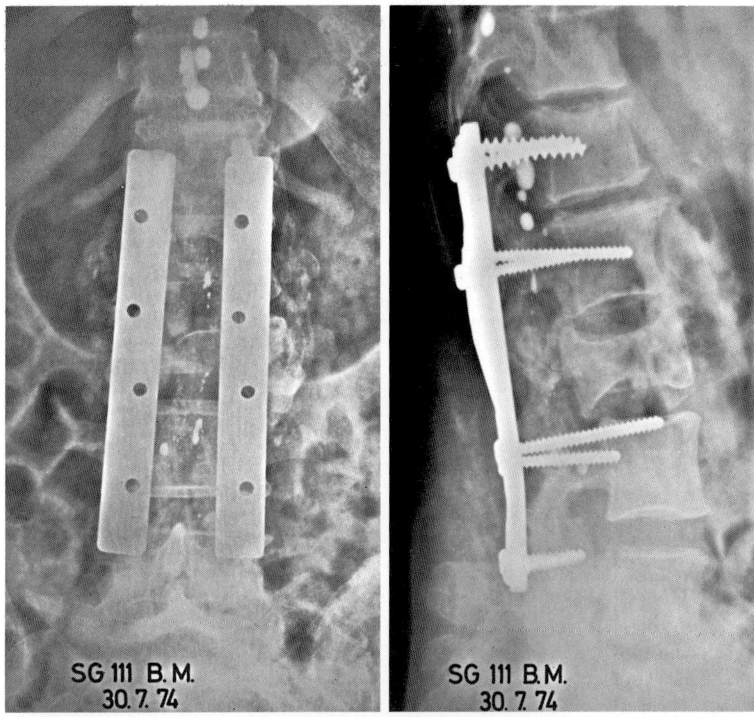

b

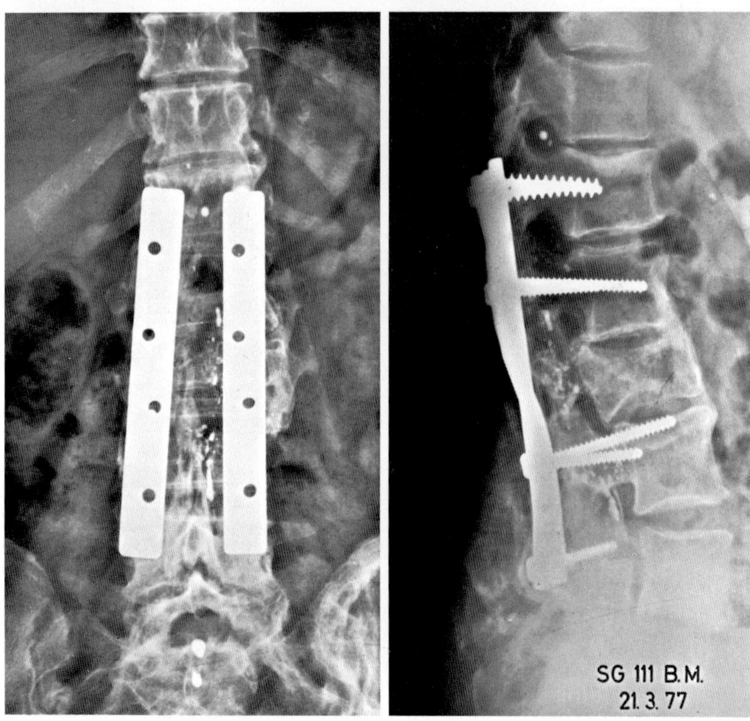

c

8 Internal Fixation Plates with a Specialized Form or Function

Form and function are interrelated in a fashion characteristic of the locomotor system. Nature attempts to create a harmony between form and function, and the science of biomechanics acknowledges this harmony as a natural principle. This principle can be utilized therapeutically in an endless variety of ways, including internal plate fixation.

8.1 Plate as Lever Arm for Bone Lengthening

Many methods are available for the lengthening of a long bone. The best method in a given case is that which achieves the purpose with a minimum of material and labor.

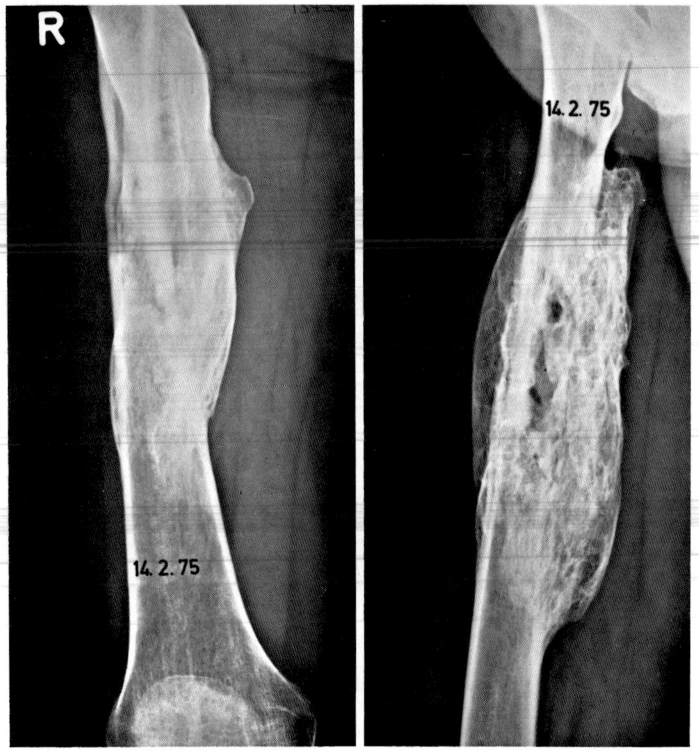

a

Example 1: Malunited femoral shaft fracture with shortening and marked callus formation (Fig. 72)

The problem: An additional 4 cm of bone length must be obtained in a single stage.

The solution: The broad plate for the proposed internal fixation is used as a lever to lengthen the bone. The length gain is maintained by applying an anti-glide plate to the anterior surface. This type of double plating, strictly prohibited in fresh fractures, is of great value in hypervascularized bone with a massive callus.

Fig. 72a–d. Plate used as lever arm in lengthening osteotomy.
H.S., ♀, age 47, No. 184860.
a Femoral fracture healed with 4-cm limb shortening; massive callus formation.
b *Plan of operation:* The plate is screwed to both fragments in such a way that when it is rotated through 150°, the desired degree of lengthening is obtained. A separate anti-glide plate is applied for additional stability.
c *Postoperative roentgenogram:* 4-cm lengthening.
d *One year after operation:* Uneventful healing of osteotomy

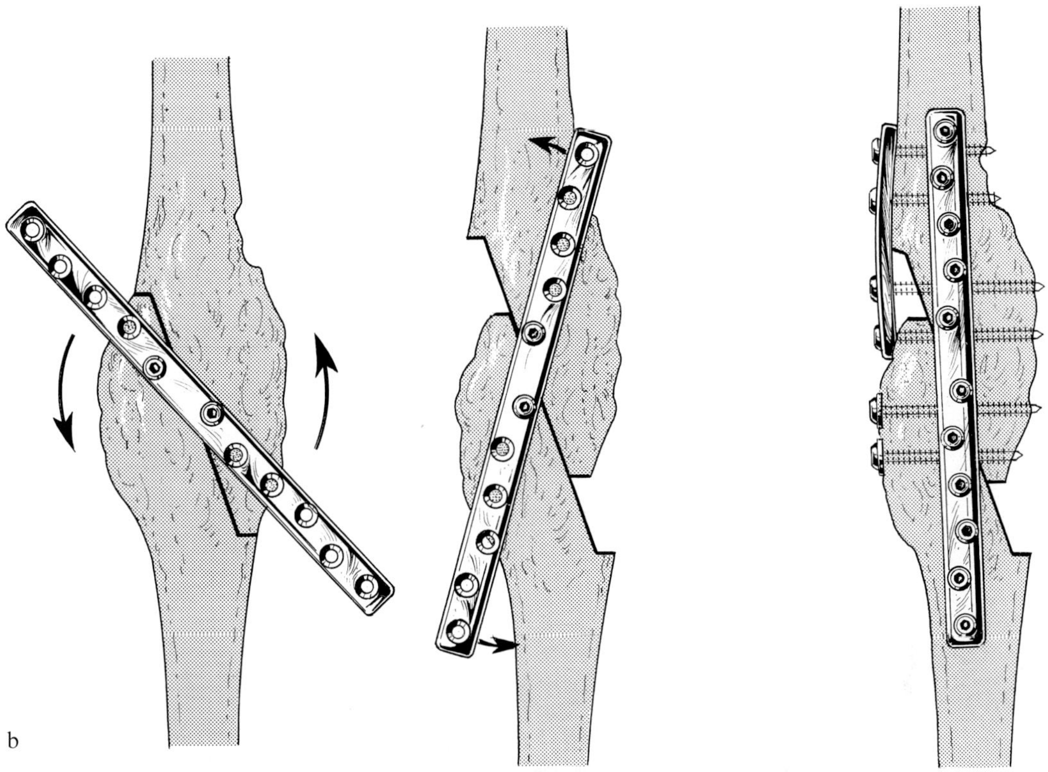

b

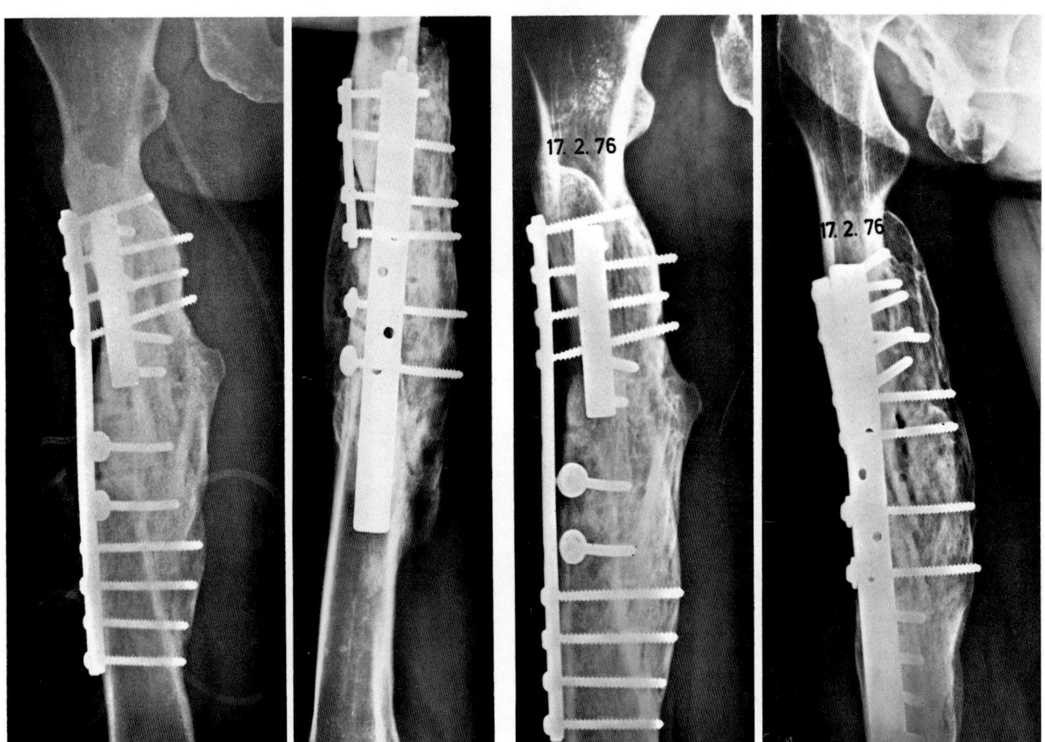

c, d

8.2 "Wave Plate"

The wave plate is a plate specially contoured to leave room for bone substance that is either left intact or has yet to be formed (by cancellous grafting).

a, b

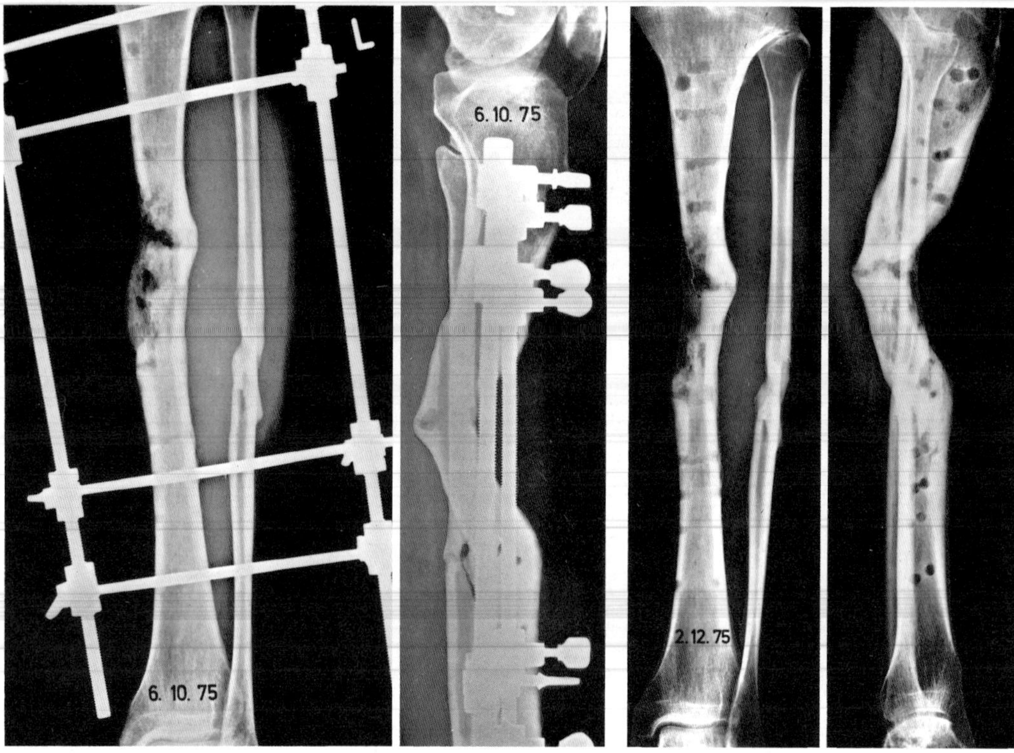

Example 1: Pseudarthrosis of the tibia after anterior saucerization and posterior bone grafting (Fig. 73)

The problem: Because of the transverse course of the pseudarthrosis, healing is prevented by the action of compressive forces anteriorly and tensile forces posteriorly.

The solution: First a wave plate is applied posteriorly to create a tension band so that the pseudarthrosis is stable. Next the bony defect left by the saucerization is filled with autologous cancellous bone to allow normal load bearing. After healing of the pseudarthrosis, the tension band plate may be removed with no danger of fatigue fracture at the former site of the pseudarthrosis.

Fig. 73a–f. Wave plate as a tension band.
F.R., ♂, age 30, No. 178947.
a Formerly open, infected tibial fracture. Status after saucerization and Thiersch grafting.
b *Pseudarthrosis:* Posterior bowing, infection healed.
c *Operative technique:* A broad plate is given a "wave" contour to serve as a tension band. A compression-resistant tibia is reconstructed by anterior cancellous grafting. The operation is done in two stages.
d *Status after second stage.*
e *Four months after operation:* Pseudarthrosis healed.
f *Two years after operation, after implant removal:* Complete recovery

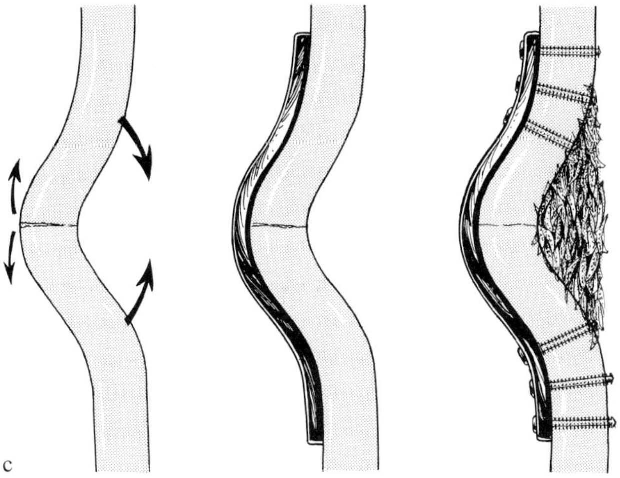

c

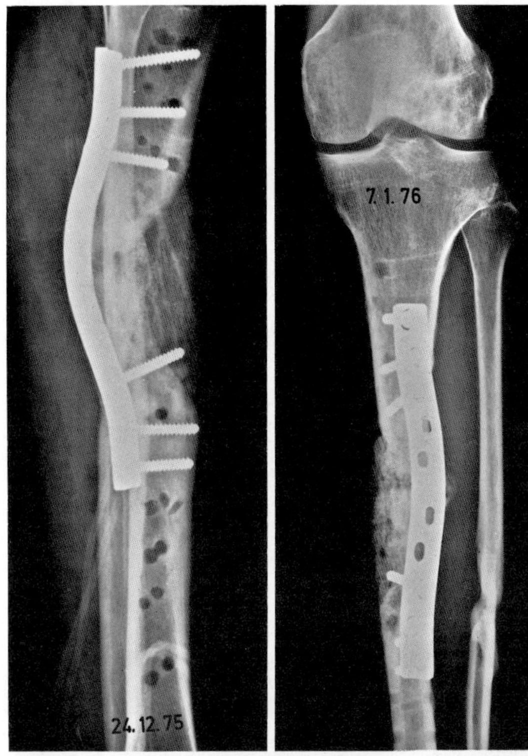

d

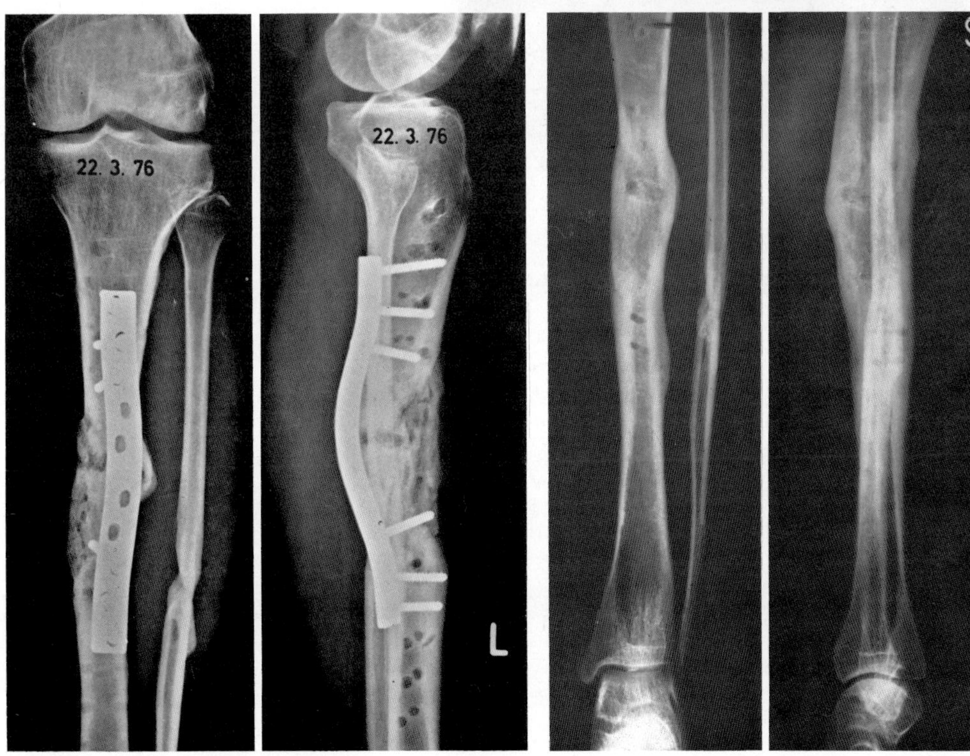

e, f

Example 2: Pseudarthrosis of the femoral shaft from necrosis of the lateral cortex (Fig. 74)

The problem: After repeated operations, necrosis persists in a portion of the lateral cortex where tension resistance is needed. As a result, the pseudarthrosis is unable to heal properly, and a refracture or fatigue fracture may occur.

The solution: It is not sufficient to apply a tension band plate alone, for ultimately this function should be exercised by living bone. This goal can be achieved with the aid of a wave plate, below which is applied a graft of cancellous bone. In this way the pseudarthrosis can go on healing even without the protection of a direct overlying tension band.

Fig. 74a–i. Wave plate used to bridge a cancellous bone graft.
G.U., ♀, age 30, No. 162903.
a Comminuted fracture of the femoral shaft.
b *Initial treatment:* Supracondylar Kirschner wire traction.
c *Initial plating:* Poor reduction, deficient medial buttress.
d *Six months after injury:* Infected pseudarthrosis.
e *Reoperation:* Debridement, repeat internal fixation, cancellous grafting.
f *Fifteen months after reoperation:* Bone necrosis still present on lateral side, predisposing to refracture.
g *Principle of wave plate:* The bone beneath the straight plate cannot be adequately revascularized. The wave plate, on the other hand, allows vascular ingrowth into the bone.
h Wave plate and cancellous graft in situ.
i *Two years and 8 months after grafting and wave-plating:* Cancellous bone incorporated; bone healthy on all sides, pseudarthrosis healed

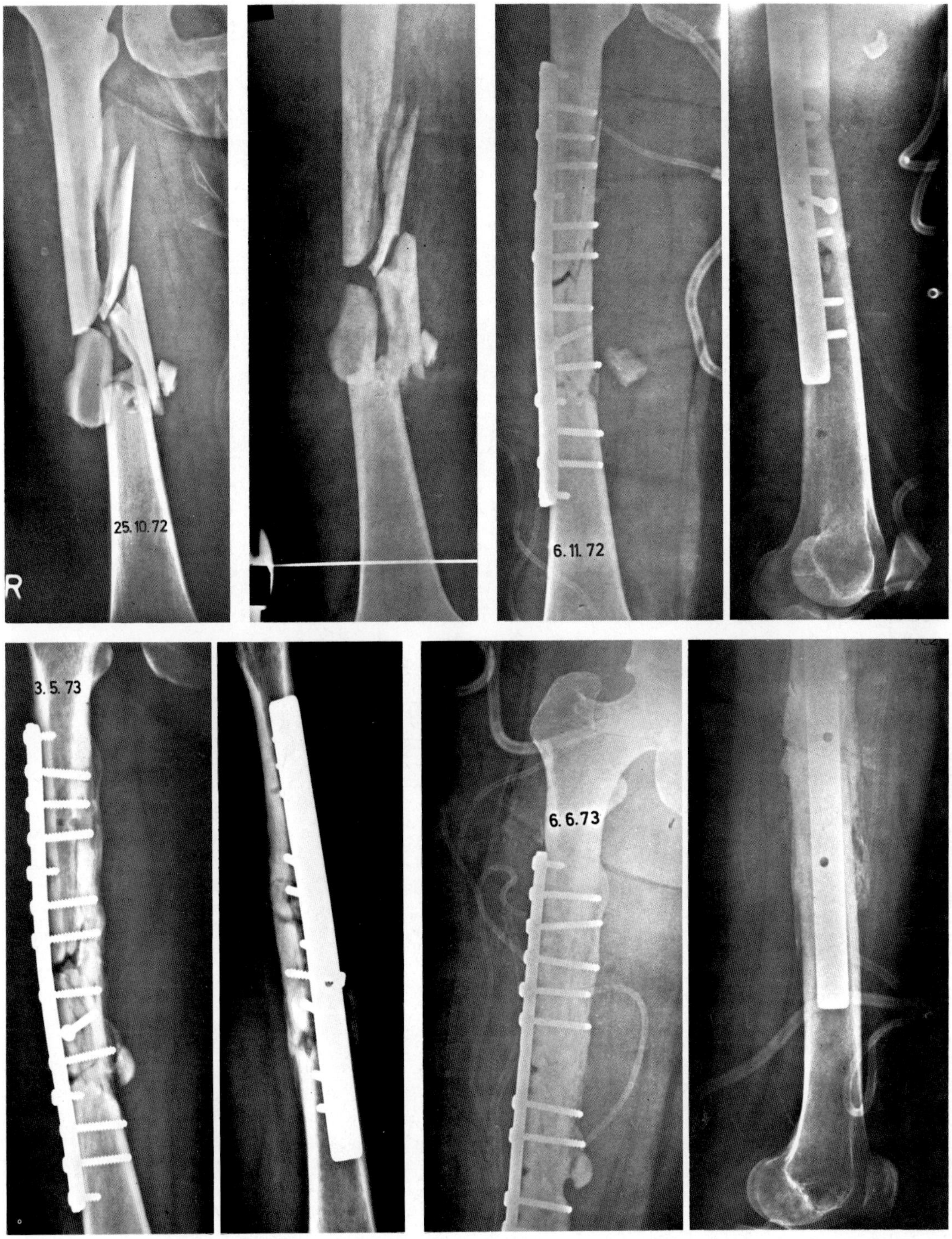

a–c

d, e

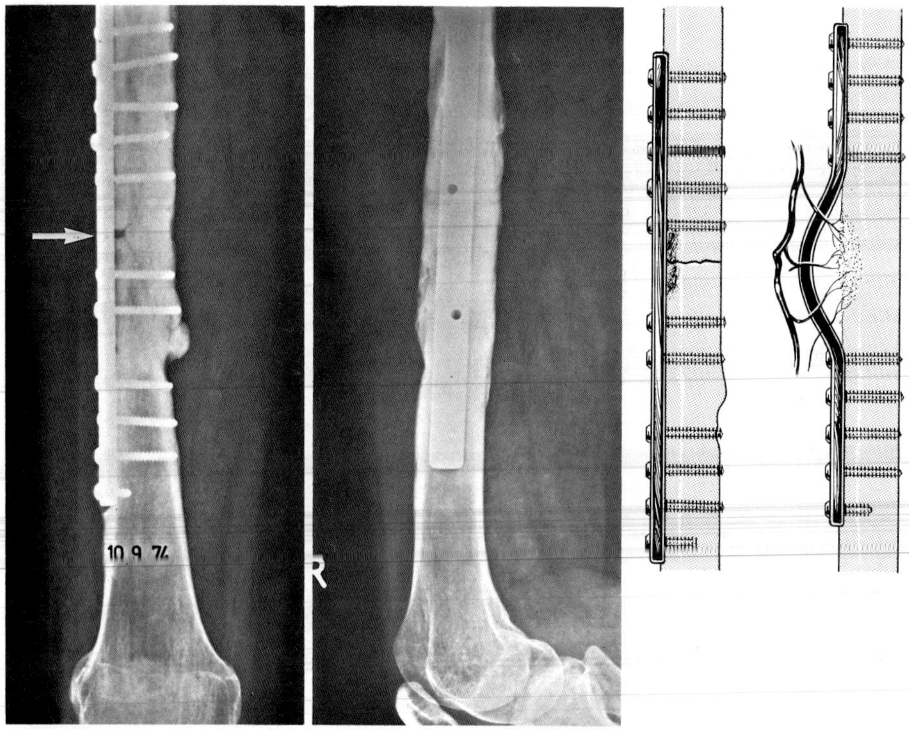

f, g

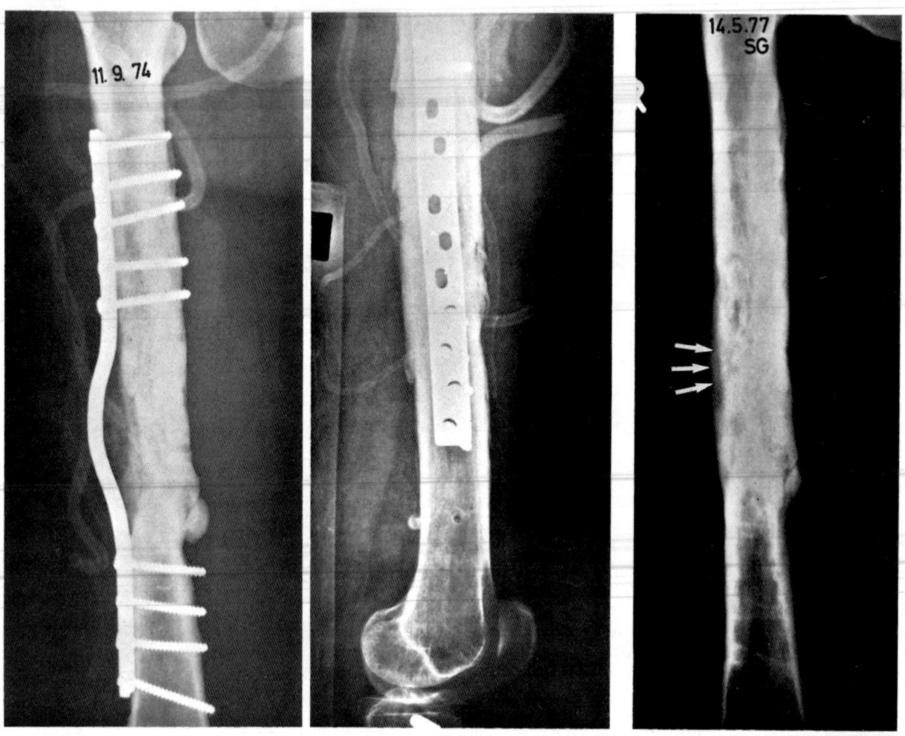

h, i

Fig. 74f–i. Legend see p. 150

8.3 Plating for Symphyseal Rupture

For the typical rupture of the symphyseal iliosacral joint, dynamic, tension-resistant internal wiring combined with postoperative bed rest is considered the treatment of choice. In fractures of the pelvic girdle with complex displacement of the fragments however, wiring of the symphysis is not sufficient.

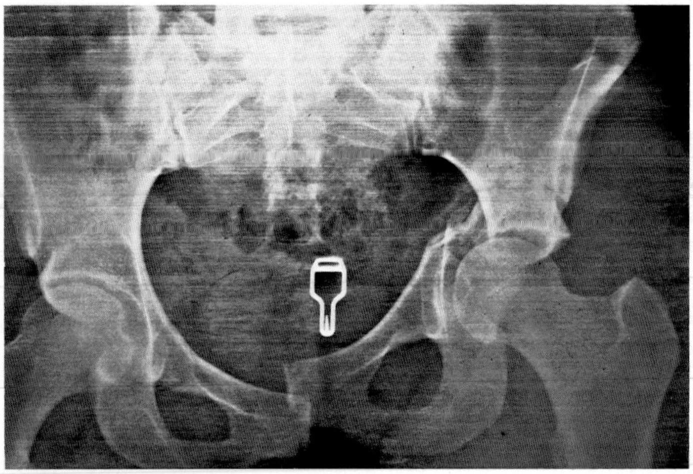

a

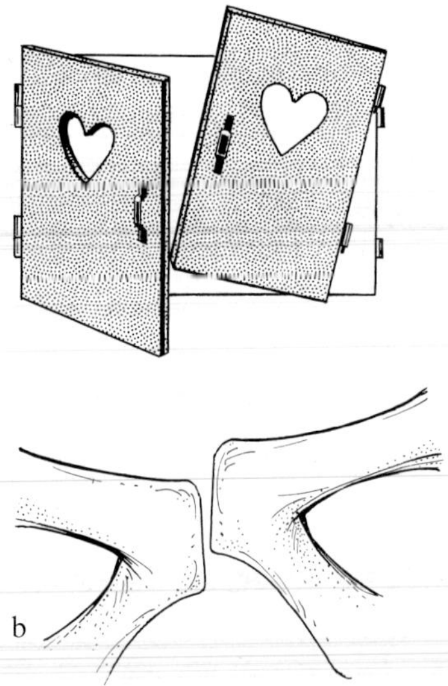

b

Example 1: Fracture of the pelvic girdle, central dislocation of the hip and symphyseal rupture (Fig. 75)

The problem: The injury is analogous to the state of a broken or an unhinged shutter with three weak points – the two hinges and the latch. A stable fixation of the symphysis contributes to a secure internal fixation of the acetabular fracture; symphyseal reduction is essential, in fact, for the congruent reduction of the intra-articular fracture.

The solution: Formerly in the operative care of these fractures the acetabular fracture was reduced and stabilized from a posterior approach only. To improve the reduction anteriorly, it has proved sufficient to free the locked symphysis in a second operation and stabilize it with a semitubular plate, a small corticocancellous iliac graft having been interposed between the two freshened rami of the symphysis. As a result, the congruity of the hip joint is improved.

Fig. 75a–g. Semitubular plate as a "latch" in symphyseal rupture. W.A.U., ♀, age 25, No. 119700.
a, b Symphyseal rupture and acetabular fracture are analogous to a shutter that has come partially unhinged.
c, d *First operation:* Posterior approach to the acetabulum, internal fixation of the posterior pillar and posterior lip; approach to iliac crest and care of cranial pillar: The "shutter" is replaced on its hinge.
e, f *Second operation:* Open reduction of the symphysis, bone graft insertion, and plate fixation. This improves the reduction of the anterior pillar: The shutter is back on its hinge and the latch is closed; the pelvic girdle is again stable.
g *Eight years after injury:* Hip joint shows no signs of arthrosis, symphysis is stable, patient is free of complaints

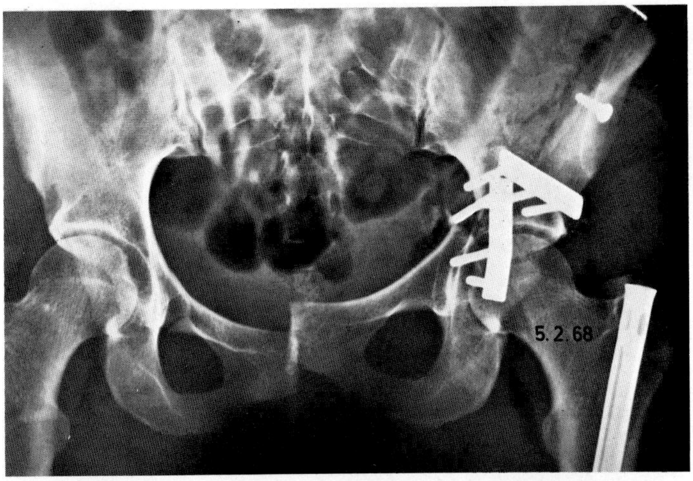

c

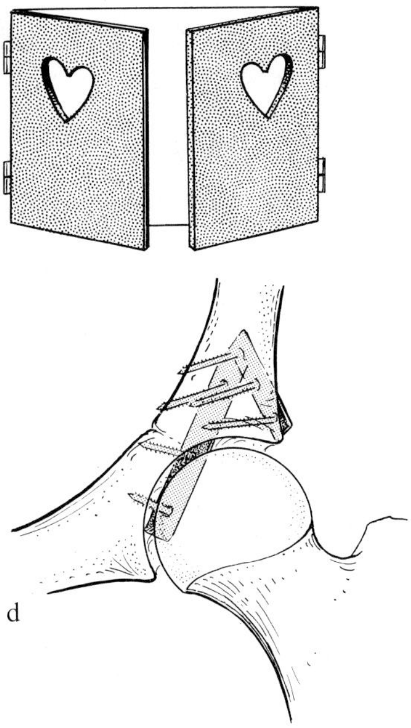

d

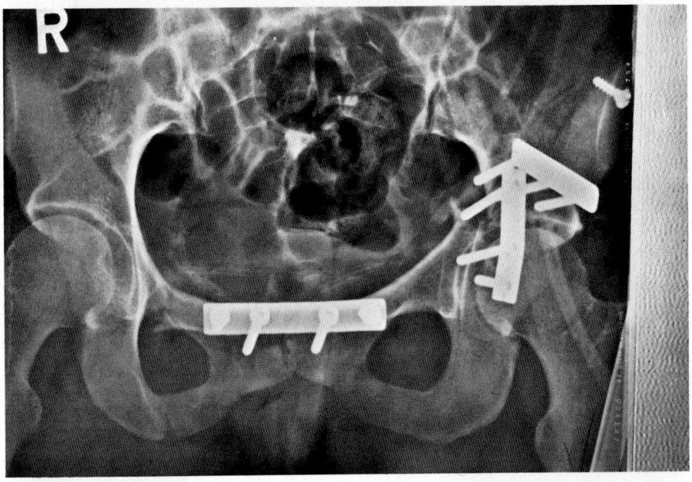

e

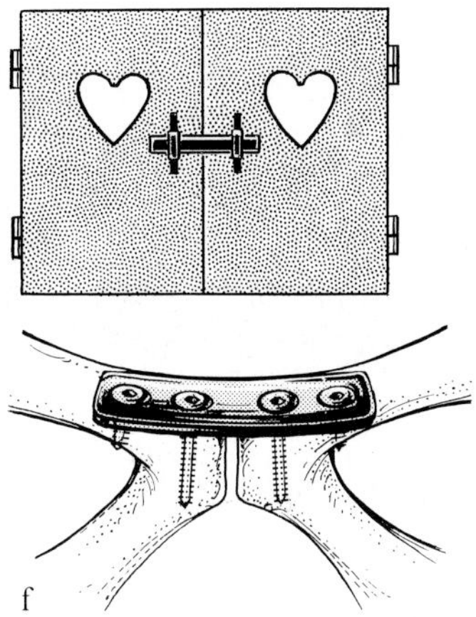

f

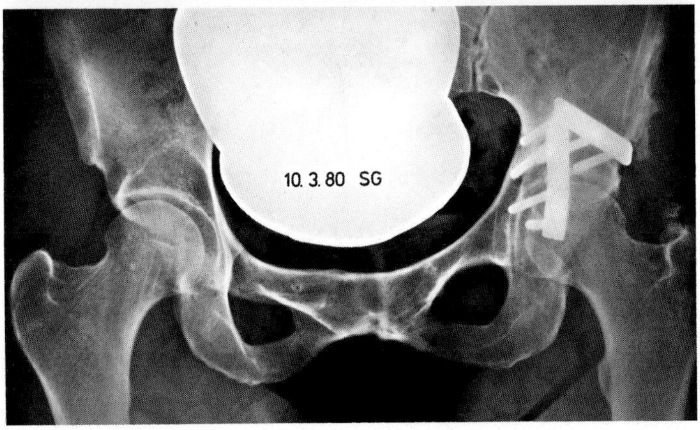

g

8.4 Semitubular Plate as a Tension Band

While some degree of elasticity is desired in the shaft of internal fixation plates, it is particularly desirable in the vicinity of the epiphysis. Here the cancellous bone often yields somewhat, and this should not be opposed by a rigid plate; otherwise loosening or breakage of the implant or pseudarthrosis could result.

a

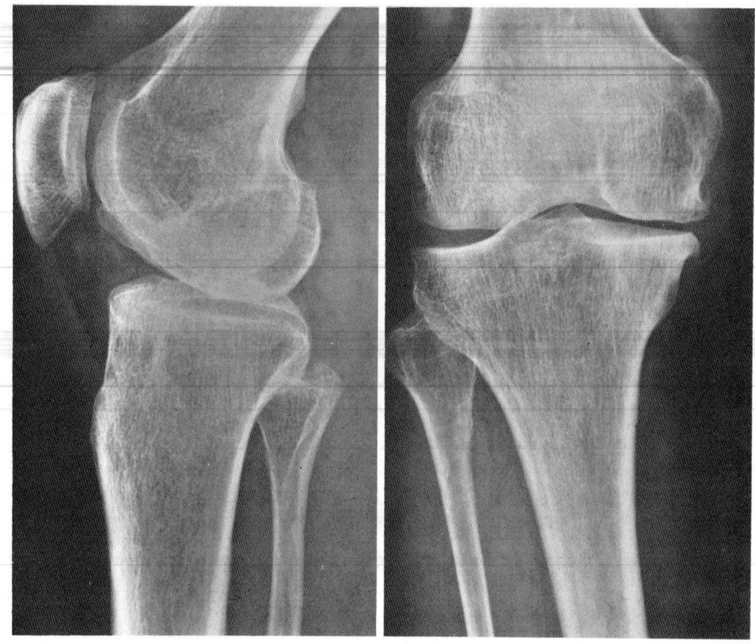

Example 1: High tibial osteotomy (Fig. 76)

The problem: In varus gonarthrosis, the upper tibial osteotomy should be fixed securely enough to permit exercise. In the event of an over- or undercorrection, moreover, it should be possible following wound healing to carry out a secondary correction in the anesthetized patient before encasing the limb in plaster.

The solution: A four- or five-hole semitubular plate is driven into the tibial head parallel to the joint space, where it will gain an excellent hold in the cancellous bone. Following the osteotomy, a lag screw is passed through the protruding plate hole and anchored in the anterior tibial border. The tension band is not rigid, but has a dynamic elasticity sufficient to allow mobilization.

Fig. 76a–d. Semitubular plate for dynamic tension banding.
G.J., ♀, age 64, No. 190712.
a Typical varus gonarthrosis.
b *Principle of operation:* The semitubular plate is driven in parallel to the joint space, and the end of the plate is bent. A lateral wedge is removed without rupturing the medial periosteum. The osteotomy is closed by tightening the oblique screw.
c *Postoperative roentgenogram.*
d *Sixteen months after operation:* Osteotomy healed, patient free of complaints.

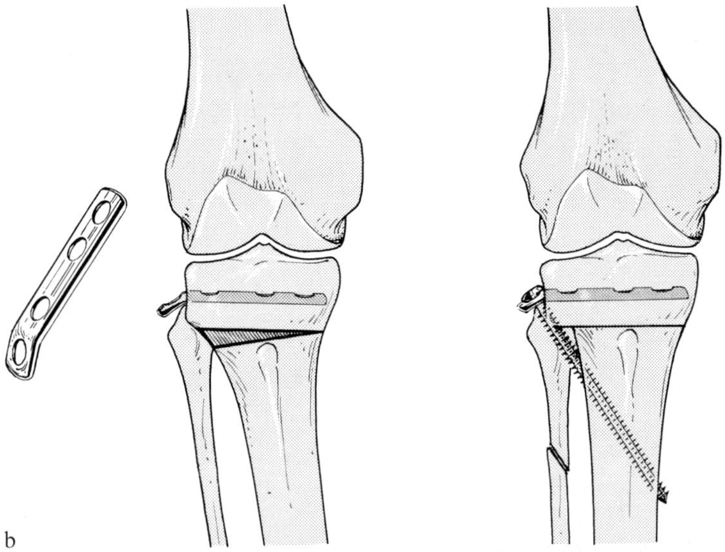

b

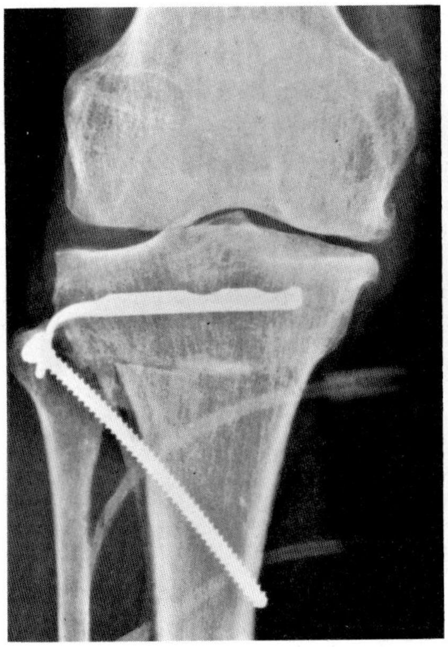

c

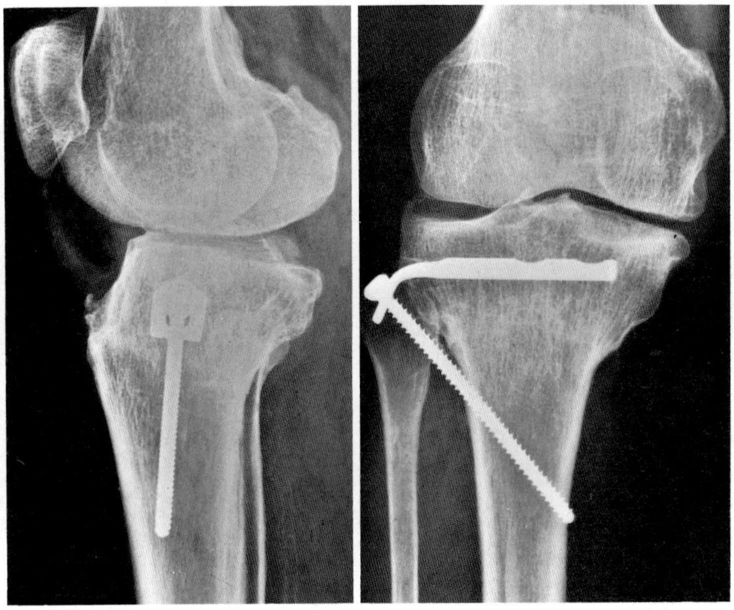

d

Example 2: Subcapital rotation osteotomy of the humerus for recurrent dislocation of the shoulder (Fig. 77)

The problem: The loose cancellous bone of the humeral head affords a dubious hold for screws and ordinary plates. For this reason wire-loop tension bands passed through the rotator cuff are generally necessary in the internal fixation of fractures.

The solution: An alternative to inserting a wire through the rotator cuff is the use of an angled blade plate fashioned intraoperatively from a six- or seven-hole semitubular plate: the longer end of the plate is hammered flat and bent to a 100° angle between two plate holes. The remainder of the plate is curved somewhat to form a "condylar plate." The plate is mounted on the lateral surface of the humeral shaft to create a tension band for stabilizing the subcapital rotation osteotomy. This "isoelastic" plate fixes the osteotomy better than any rigid plate.

Fig. 77 a–d. Semitubular plate as a tension-band condylar plate.
N.T., ♀, age 25, No. 180334.
a Recurrent shoulder dislocation with typical Hill-Sachs lesion.
b *Semitubular plate as a condylar plate:* The plate has to be constructed by the surgeon and is securely anchored in the humeral head.
c *Two months after operation:* Osteotomy is healed and stable on loading.
d *One year after operation:* Osteotomy line is obliterated

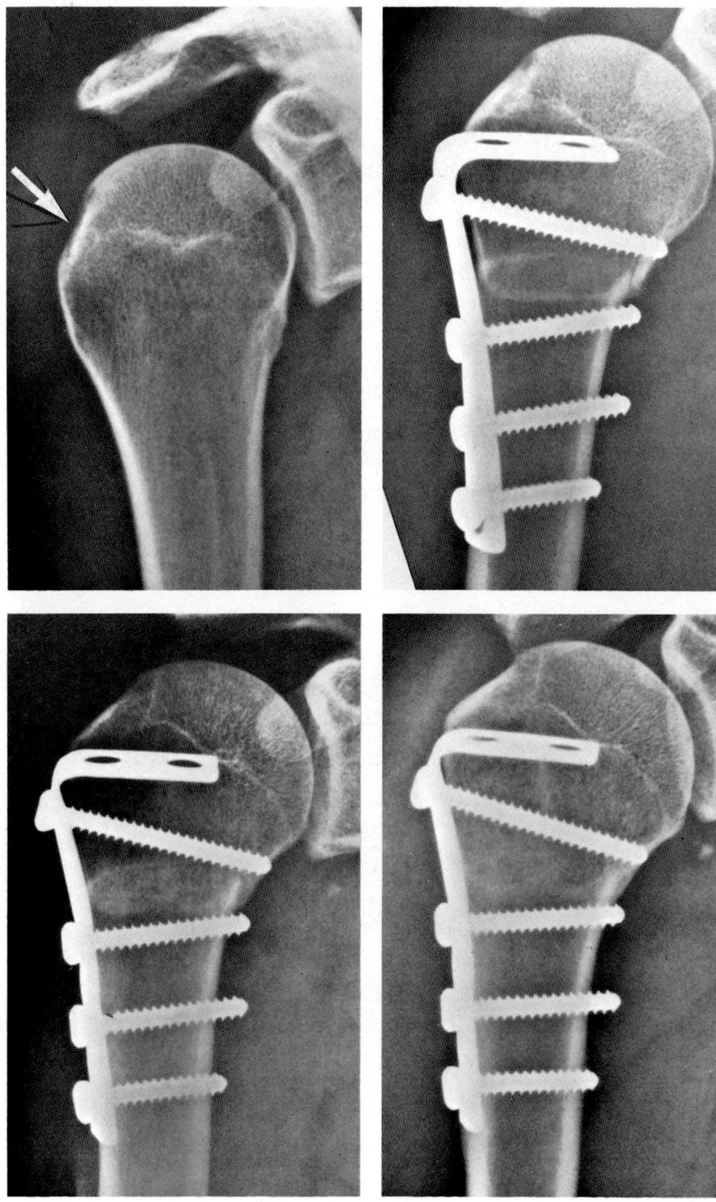

a, b

c, d

8.5 "Biological" Fixation of the Fractured Tibia

In comminuted fractures, particularly severely comminuted fractures of the tibia with multiple small fragments, it must be decided whether it is prudent to perform a complete internal fixation in which the periosteum of numerous fragments would have to be sacrificed. To avoid jeopardizing the vitality of the fragments further, therefore, one might elect for a less-than-complete reconstruction. We call this type of internal fixation biological, because it relies heavily upon biological mechanisms of repair.

a–c

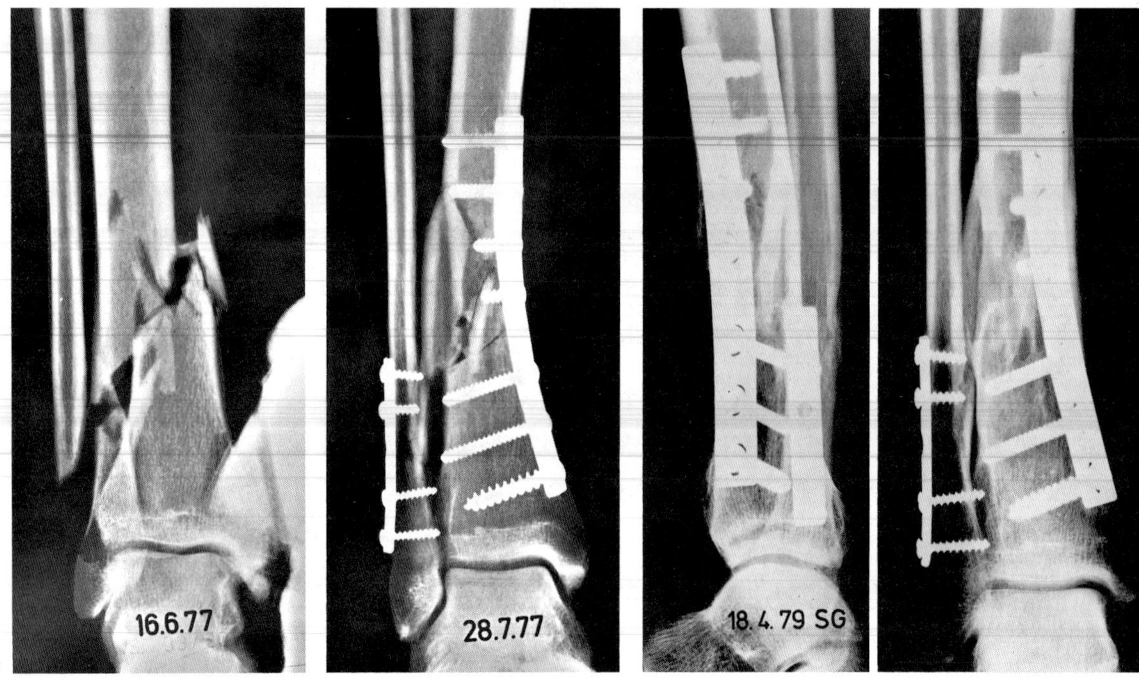

Example 1: Fracture of the tibia and fibula with comminution of the distal third of the tibia (Fig. 78)

The problem: Unless an accurate reduction is carried out, the limb will not be sufficiently stable for postoperative mobilization, one of the main purposes of internal fracture fixation thus being defeated.

The solution: Open reduction to correct the length and the angular and rotational alignment is carried out only on the medial side of the tibia and is secured with a medial plate. No effort is made to locate the lateral fragments; these are left in place to become reincorporated as grafts. To improve the stability of this arrangement, the fibula is also plated. It is this plate which chiefly obviates the need for lateral tibial fixation.

Fig. 78a–c. Biological internal fixation. S.M., ♂, age 32, No. 208969.
a Comminuted fracture of the distal tibia.
b *Operation:* Internal fixation of the fibula with one-third tubular plate; fixation of the tibia is limited to reconstruction of the medial side and appositional fixation with a relatively short plate. The small fragments are not disturbed and are left attached to the periosteum as "pedicle grafts."
c *Twenty-two months after injury:* Complete recovery. The lateral "autologous" tibial graft is well integrated

8.6 Buttressed Angled Blade Plate for the Proximal Femur

Internal fixations of the proximal femur must follow the principle of the medial buttress, i. e., compression-resistant bone combined with a tension-resistant implant. In the surgery of tumors, the medial bony buttress is often deficient.

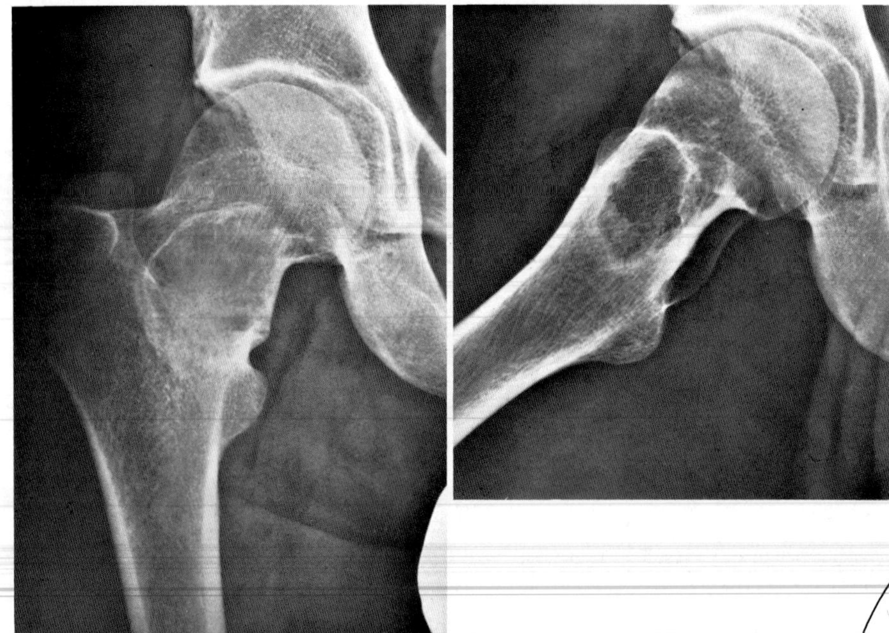

a

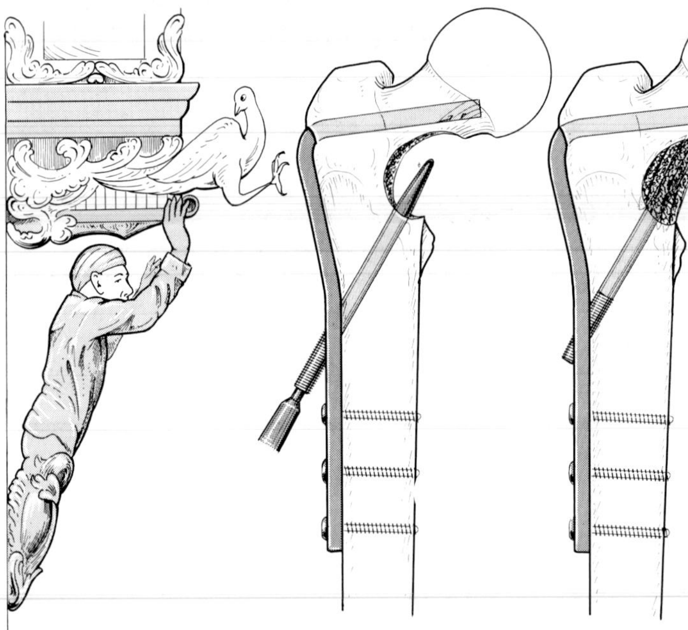

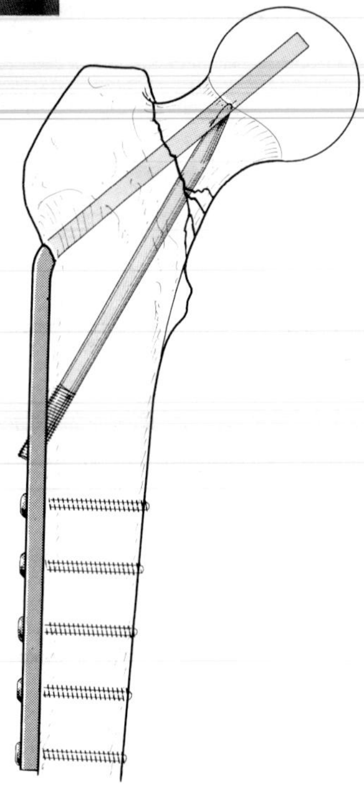

b

Fig. 79a–e. Buttressed angled blade plate (condylar or 130° plate) in a femoral neck tumor.
G.P., ♂, age 29, No. 197378.
a The fibroma has penetrated the calcar, with a very great risk of spontaneous fracture.
b *Principle of operation:* Just as the balcony is supported by the "Atlas," the angled blade is supported by a threaded pin, its tip resting in a groove in the plate blade. Either the condylar or 130° plate may be used; the latter is shown for the case of a comminuted femoral neck fracture (*4*).(WEISSMANN and SALAMA)

Example 1: Fibroma of the femoral neck with erosion of the calcar (Fig. 79)

The problem: The medial bony buttress is destroyed by resection of the tumor.

The solution: After the tumor resection, the calcarine defect is repaired with corticocancellous bone chips. The femoral neck is fixed with a buttressed angled blade plate, and the defect is filled with autologous cancellous bone. The buttress pin prevents varus deformity and plate breakage.

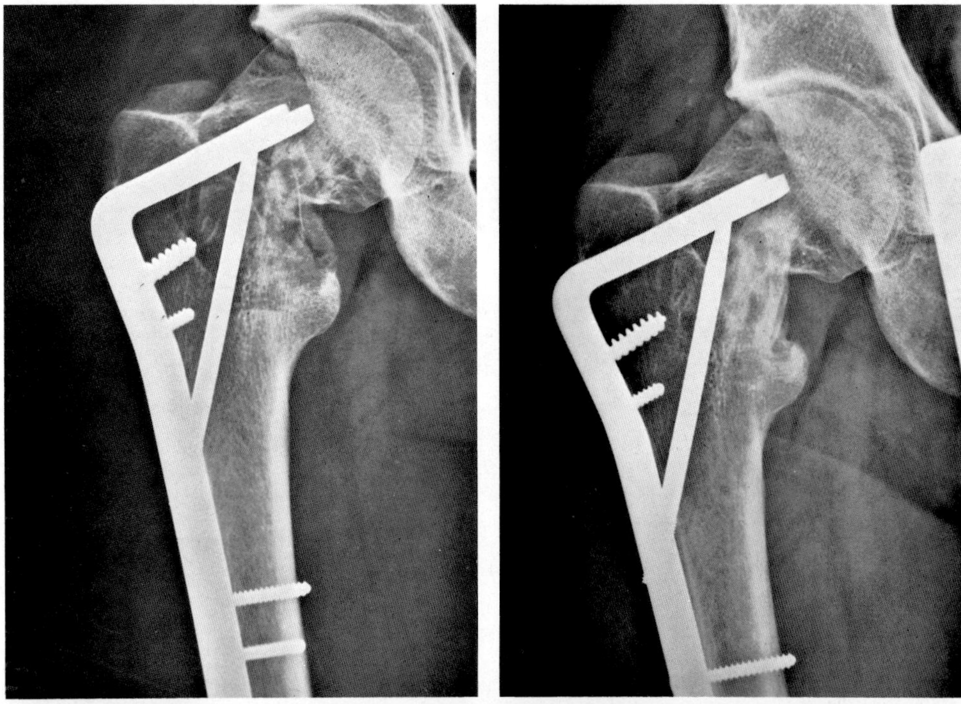

c, d

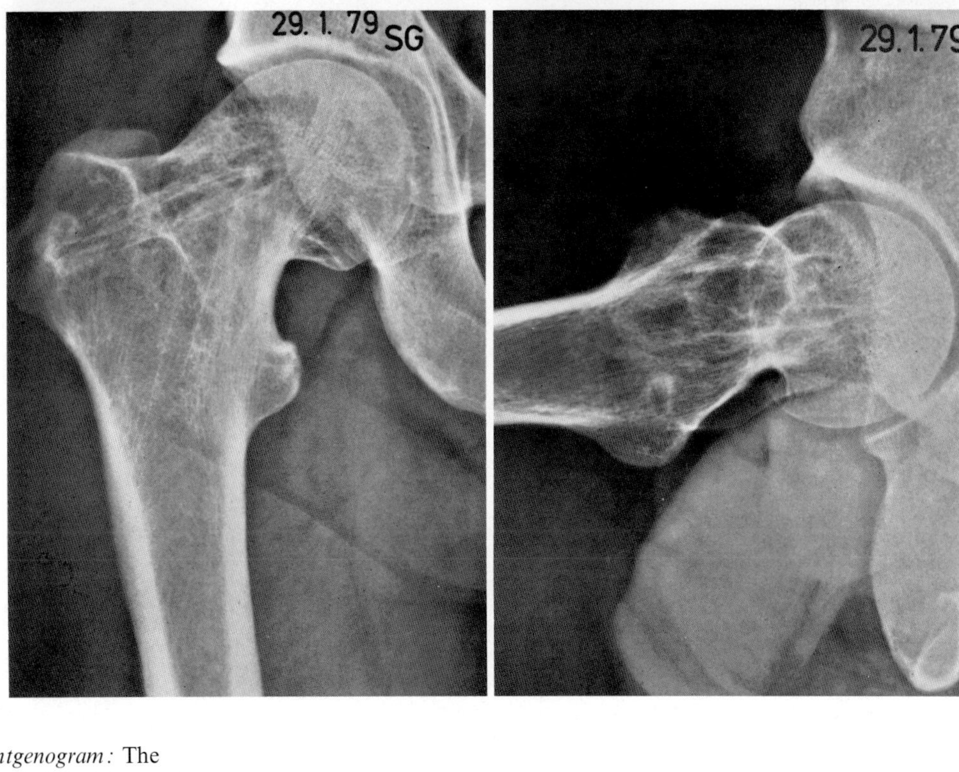

e

c *Postoperative roentgenogram:* The bone defect has been filled with autologous cancellous bone after insertion of the buttress pin.
d *Nine months after operation:* Calcar is restored.
e *Three years after operation, after implant removal:* Complete recovery

Example 2: Subtrochanteric fibrous dysplasia with weakening of the lateral and medial cortex (Fig. 80)

The problem: Following radical tumor resection, it is necessary to restore the compressive and tensile strength of the femur.

The solution: Even before the tumor resection, the condylar plate is inserted to retain the femoral shape. Then the tumor is radically excised, and the buttress pin is inserted. The lateral tension band is reinforced with a wire looped over the greater trochanter. The defect is filled with autologous cancellous bone.

Fig. 80a–c. Buttressed angled blade plate in fibrous dysplasia of the proximal femur.
S.H., ♂, age 32, No. 215600.
a The fibrous dysplasia involves both the per- and subtrochanteric areas of the proximal femur.
b *Operation:* Tumor resection, insertion of a plate buttressed with a pin. Tension banding with plate and wire loop over trochanter. Autologous bone grafting.
c *Twenty-six months after operation:* Full weight-bearing capability has been restored

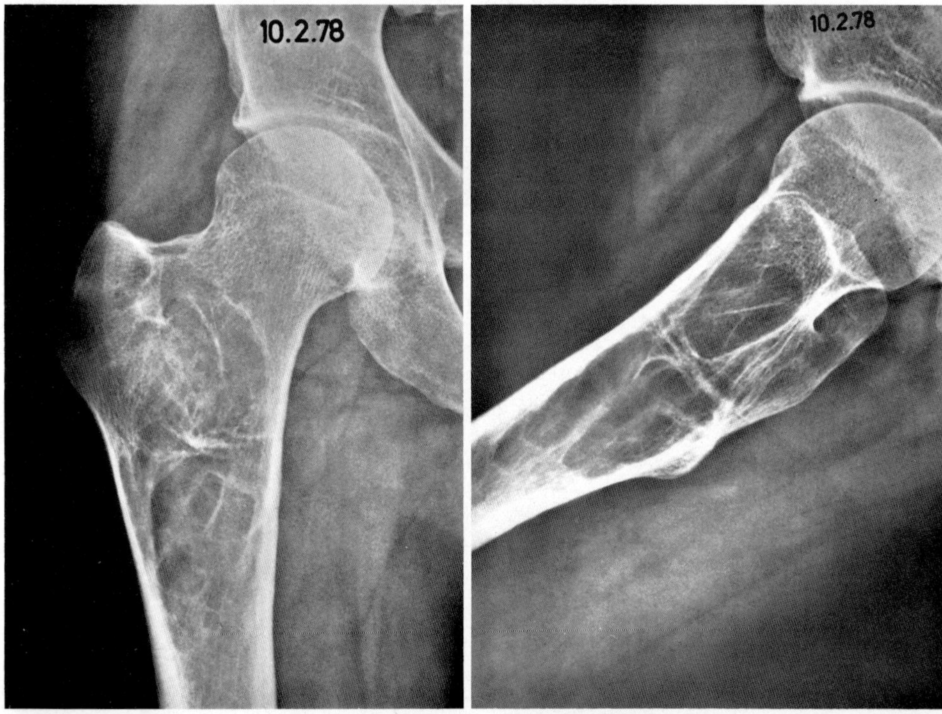

a

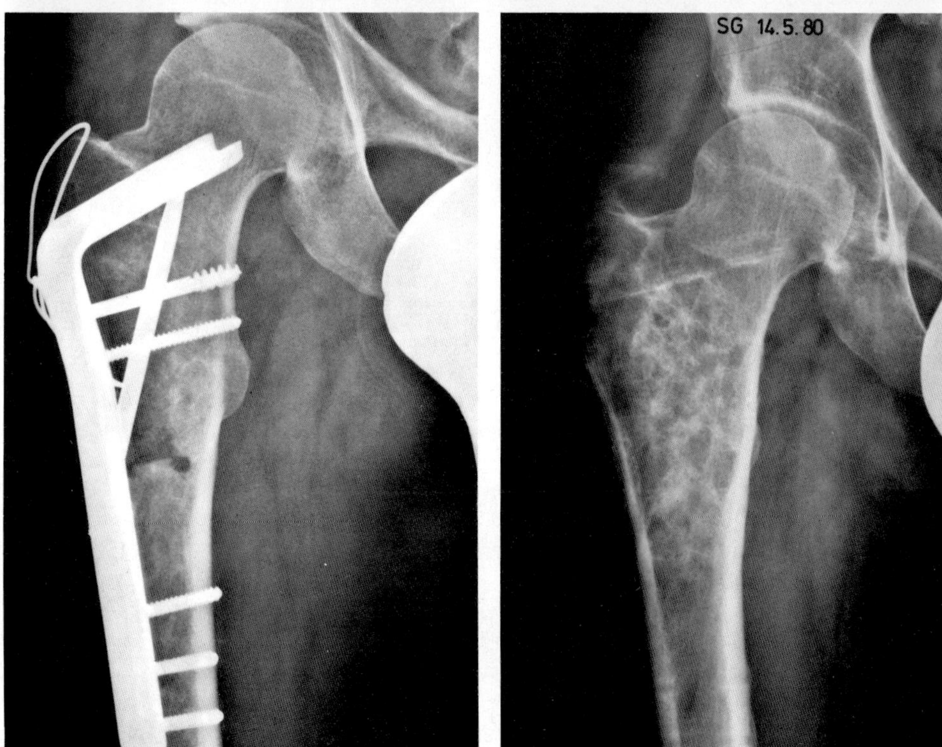

b, c

9 Medullary Nail

Occasionally a problem arises that can be solved neither by ordinary intramedullary nailing, nor by any other internal fixation method. Unusual indication and operative technique for medullary nailing may be helpful.

9.1 Medullary Nailing Combined with Bone Cement

The technique of composite plate fixation for severe osteoporosis of the proximal femur and for pathologic fractures has been described in the *Manual of Internal Fixation* (MULLER et al., 1979). A different composite fixation is presented here.

Example 1: Fracture of the proximal third of the tibia in an elderly female (Fig. 81)

The problem: It is important that the patient, an elderly woman, be mobilized again as rapidly as possible. The peripheral circulation is poor, and plating of the medial side of the tibia is therefore contraindicated. There is a danger, moreover, that internal fixation with a plate would not be very stable under loading.

The solution: After exposure of the fracture, sparing curettage of the medullary cavity in the fracture area, and anatomic reduction, the cortical bone of the proximal fragment is fenestrated on the medial side. The tibial tuberosity is opened in standard fashion, followed by the trial insertion of a thin medullary nail. The nail is then removed, the medullary cavity filled with bone cement through the cortical opening, and the nail immediately reinserted. After the cement has hardened, the fracture is stable on loading. Overall form is maintained by the cement, and axial stability by the nail.

Fig. 81 a–c. Composite internal fixation with a tibial medullary nail and bone cement.
F.K., ♀, age 79, No. 55442.
a Proximal oblique fracture in patient with senile osteoporosis.
b *Medullary nail-bone cement composite.* (Arrows indicate cortical opening for applying the cement.)
c *Five months after injury:* The fracture has healed without complications. The patient has placed full weight on the limb since the first postoperative days

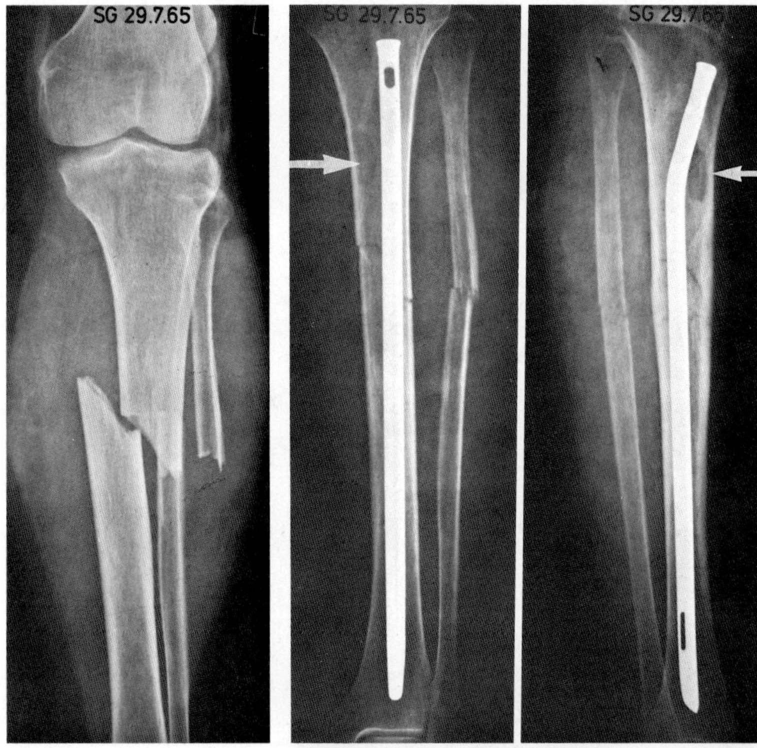

a, b

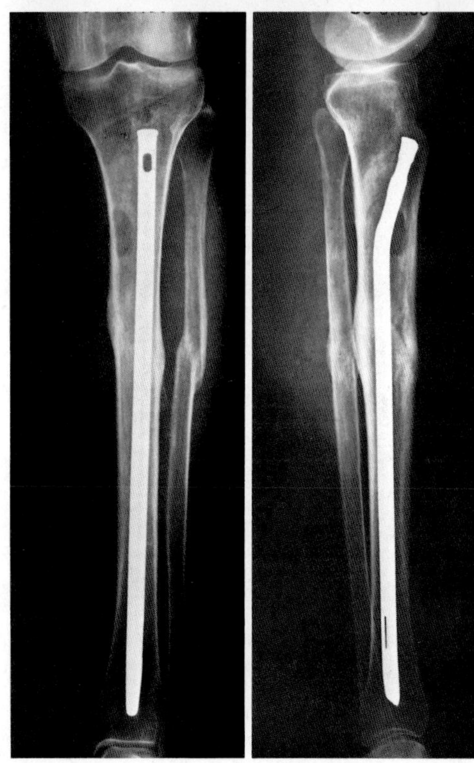

c

9.2 Distal-to-Proximal Medullary Nailing

"Retrograde" medullary nailing is indicated only in cases where normal nailing is impossible, a different method is inadvisable, and an internal fixation is nonetheless desirable.

Example 1: Fracture of the distal tibia and fibula with severe skin contusions (Fig. 82)

The problem: There are severe skin contusions of the lower leg in all areas where skin incisions would be required for normal nailing (tibial tuberosity) or plating (fracture site). The distal fragment is too short for the external fixator. The skin of the lower limb is intact in only two places – over the malleoli.

The solution. Closed nailing (i.e., without medullary reaming) is performed through two stab incisions over the malleoli with an 8-mm nail and an Oberholzer nail.

Fig. 82a–d. Retrograde route for medullary nailing of the tibia. K.M., ♂, age 29, No. 119809.
a Transverse distal fracture, skin crushed about the limb circumference from the level of the fracture to the knee. The skin is intact only over the malleoli.
b *Operation:* Small incision over both malleoli and closed nailing, with Oberholzer nail inserted laterally and 8-mm tibial nail inserted medially.
c *Ten weeks after injury:* Skin lesions healed, bone healing progressing well.
d *Sixteen months after injury:* Bone and soft tissues healed

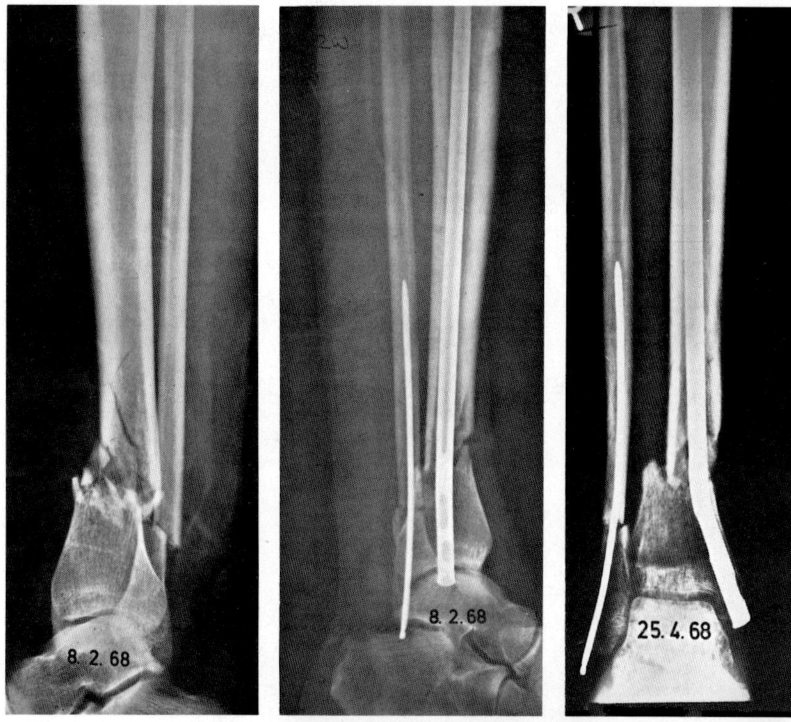

a–c

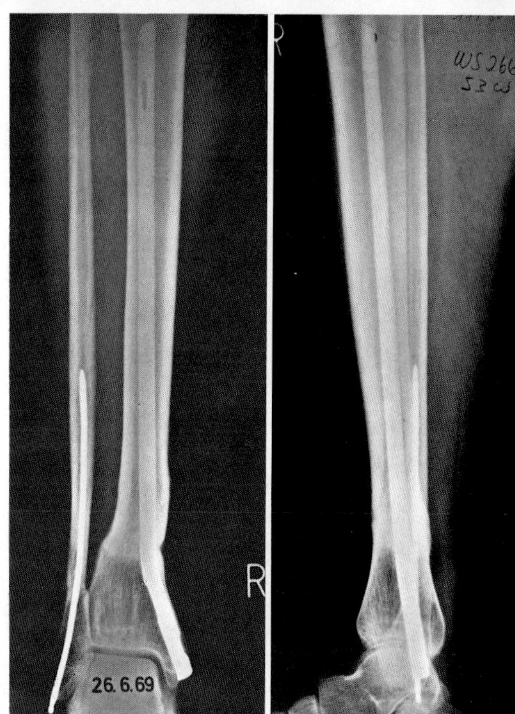

d

Example 2: Pathologic femoral fracture with radiation damage to the skin over the greater trochanter (Fig. 83)

The problem: The usual approach to the medullary cavity via the greater trochanter is not advised, because the skin there is grossly damaged as a result of radiation therapy.

The solution: The nail is inserted through the knee along the patellar ligament from the intercondylar fossa.

Fig. 83a–c. Transarticular nailing of the femur from the intercondylar fossa. S.D., ♀, age 58, No. 140991.
a *Pathologic fracture:* Metastatic tumors from mammary carcinoma, condition after irradiation of the trochanteric region; local skin is atrophic.
b *Operation:* Closed medullary nailing is carried out through the knee joint.
c *One month after operation:* Patient is again able to walk

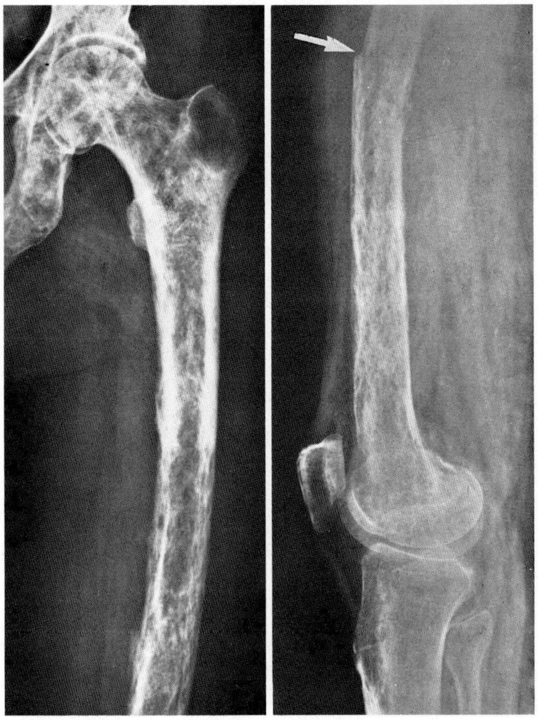

a, b

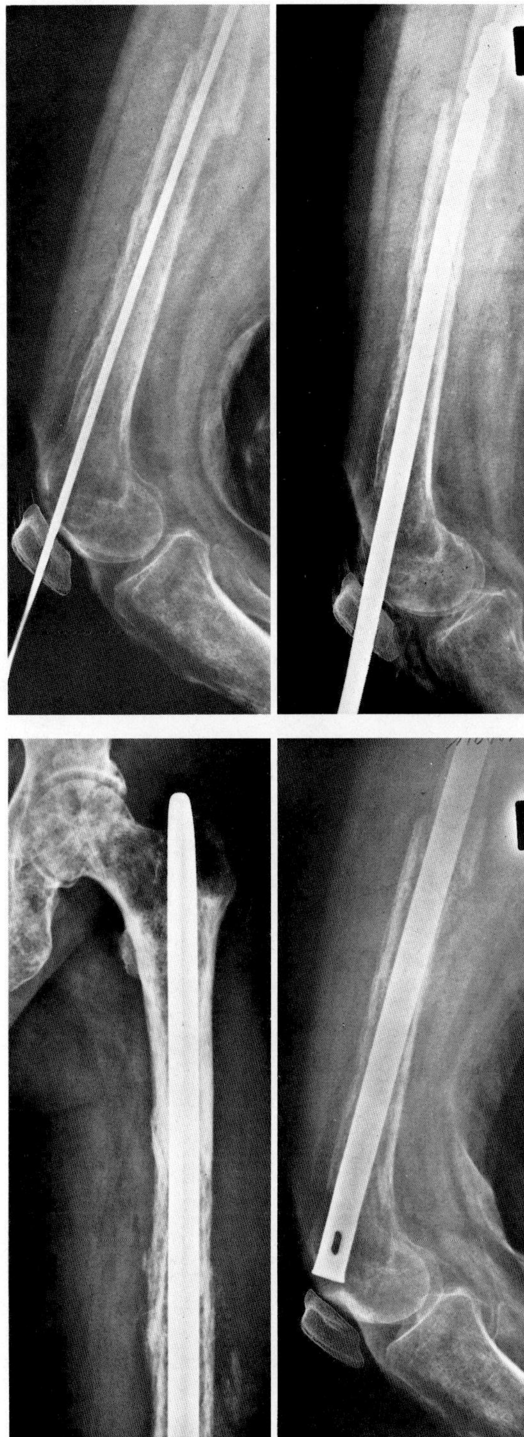

c

10 External Fixator

The classic indications for the external fixator are compression arthrodeses (Charnley) and certain open fractures (Hoffmann). Like the medullary nail, the external fixator can be useful in unusual situations by virtue of its special indications and operative technique.

10.1 Neutralization by Means of the External Fixator

The main advantage of the external fixator in the treatment of open fractures is its ability to immobilize the soft parts and promote their healing owing to its indirect stabilization of the fracture. This contributes much to the prevention of infection and, indirectly, to the healing of the fracture. An accurate reduction of the fracture facilitates revascularization of the medullary cavity, which in turn is important for keeping the fragments well perfused and free from infection. Unfortunately, the external fixator alone is incapable of providing a reduction and stability equal to that afforded by plates and screws. Nevertheless, its advantages can be utilized if its role is limited to supplementing minimal internal fixations as a means of neutralizing disruptive forces (comparable to the neutralization plate).

Example 1: Open tibial fracture (Fig. 84)

The problem: The tibial fracture is situated so far distally that the distal fragment is too short for stabilization by means of the external fixator alone.

The solution: A single lag screw is placed to obtain an anatomic reduction, thus promoting fracture healing. The external fixator neutralizes harmful forces to create optimum conditions for healing of the soft tissues and bone.

Fig. 84a–d. External fixator used for neutralization in minimal internal fixation.
B.K., ♀, age 56, No. 179491.
a Second-degree open fracture of the distal tibia: Distal fragment is too small for fixation solely by means of the external fixator.
b *Operation:* The minimal internal fixation (a single screw) is protected by the external fixator.
c *Technique:* Lag-screw fixation, debridement of wound. External fixator is applied to the tibia and metatarsus to neutralize movements about the ankle joint.
d *Ten months after injury:* Fracture and soft tissues are healed

a–c

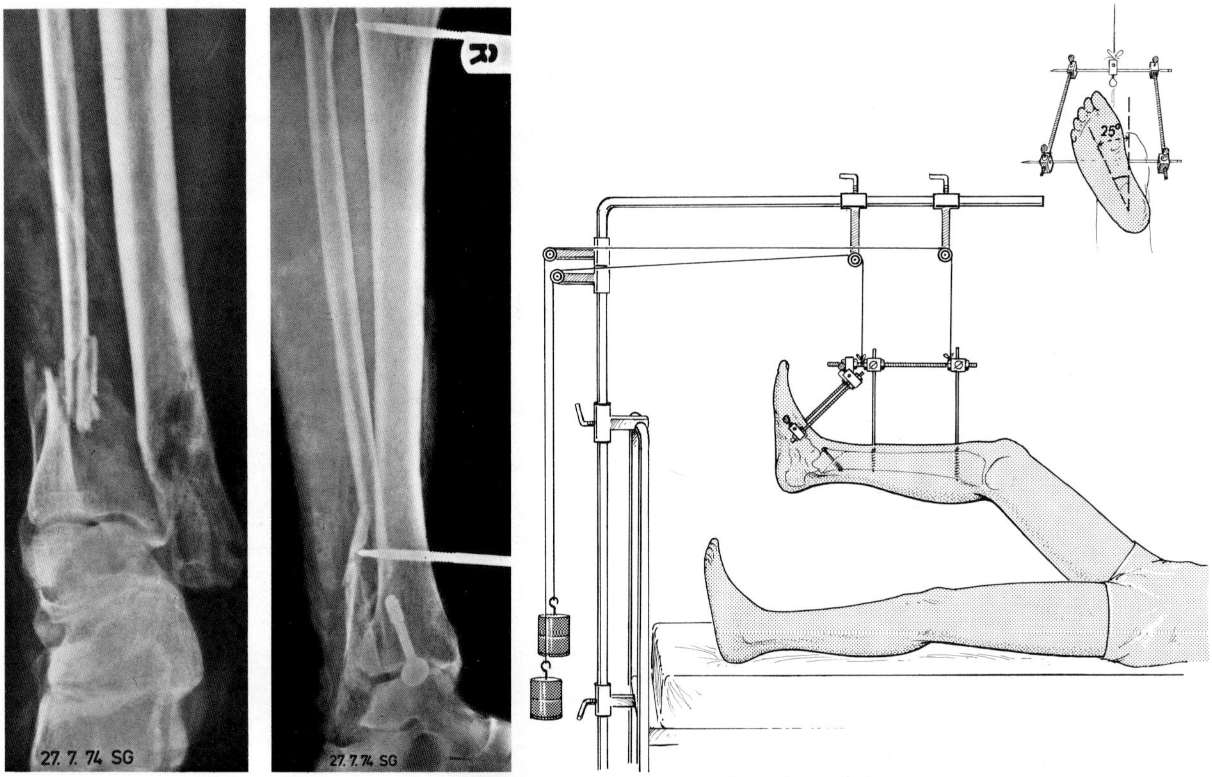

d

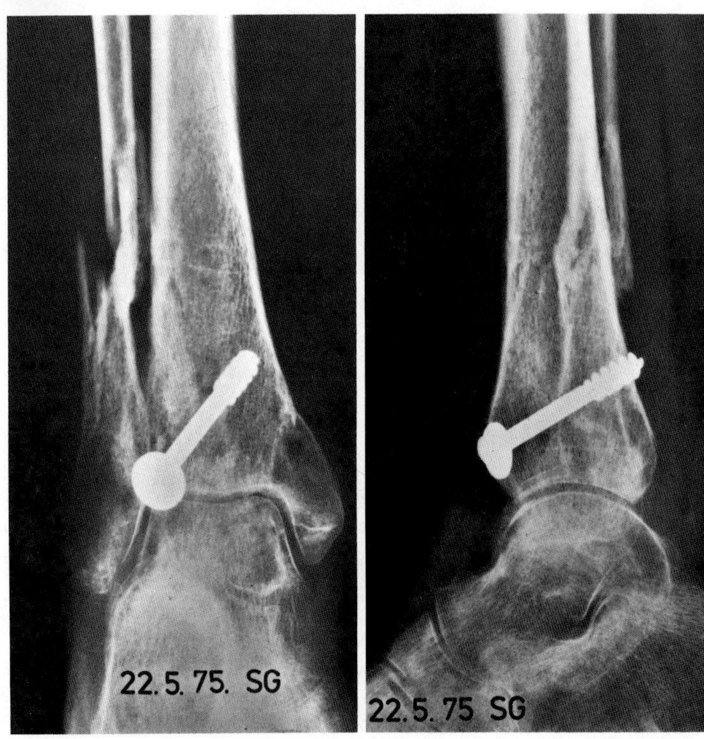

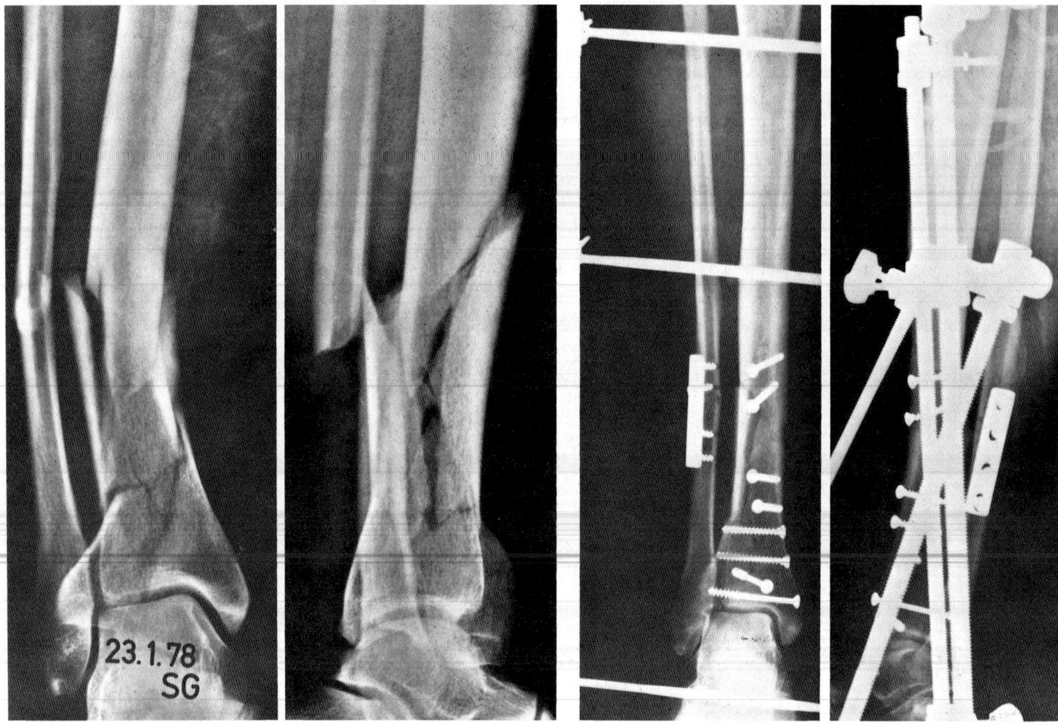

a, b

Example 2: Open tibial fracture (Fig. 85)

The problem: By means of the external fixator alone, it is impossible to approximate the fragments in their correct anatomic relation. The result is a significant amount of dead space, which can predispose to infection or malunion.

The solution: After debridement of the widely open fracture, a minimal, appositional internal fixation is undertaken to reduce or eliminate the dead space, especially between the fragments. A neutralization external fixator is then applied to protect the nonpermanent internal fixation.

Fig. 85a–e. Minimal internal fixation supplemented by external fixator. S.T., ♀, age 43, No. 215057.
a Third-degree open intra-articular comminuted fracture of the distal tibia.
b *Operation:* Wound debridement, minimal screw fixation with tibial reconstruction, external fixator applied to tibia and foot.
c *Five weeks after injury:* Reduction stable.
d *Five months after injury:* Treatment continued in below-knee walking cast.
e *One year after injury:* Soft tissues and fracture healed without complications

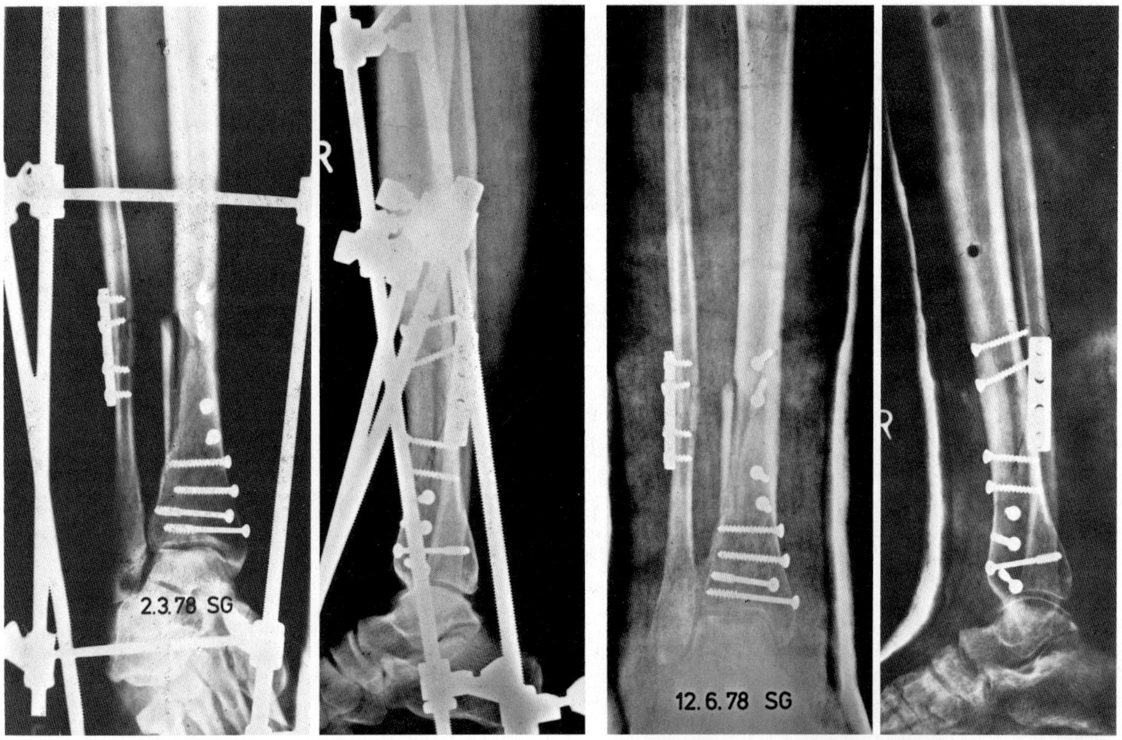

c, d

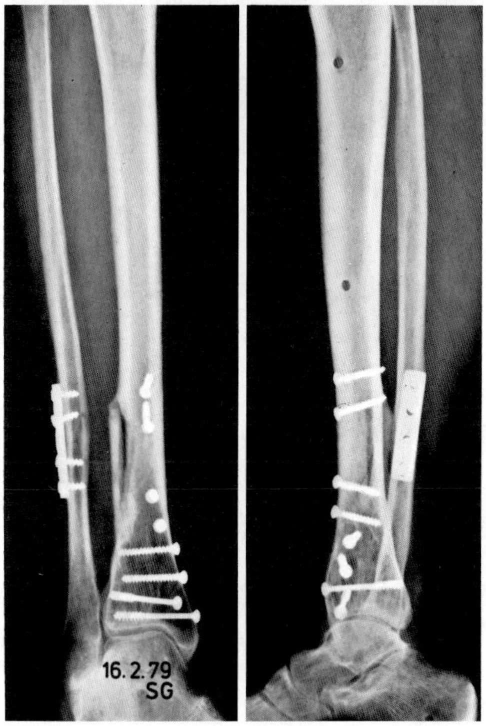

e

10.2 Special Techniques Using the External Fixator

There are two basic types of external fixator: the clamp type (Lambotte, Judet) and the frame type (Charnley). Either type may be used for fixation without compression (Hoffmann), for compression (Judet, Charnley), or for distraction (Anderson, Wagner). To prevent the clamp-type fixator from slipping, the metal pins are threaded so that they can be screwed into the bone (Schanz screws). Forces outside the longitudinal axis (compression, distraction) are difficult to transmit to the bone by means of the external fixator.

Below are examples of two special techniques with the external fixator – one for "stress-locking" the Steinmann pins to keep them from slipping in the bone, the other for applying compression in a transverse direction.

a 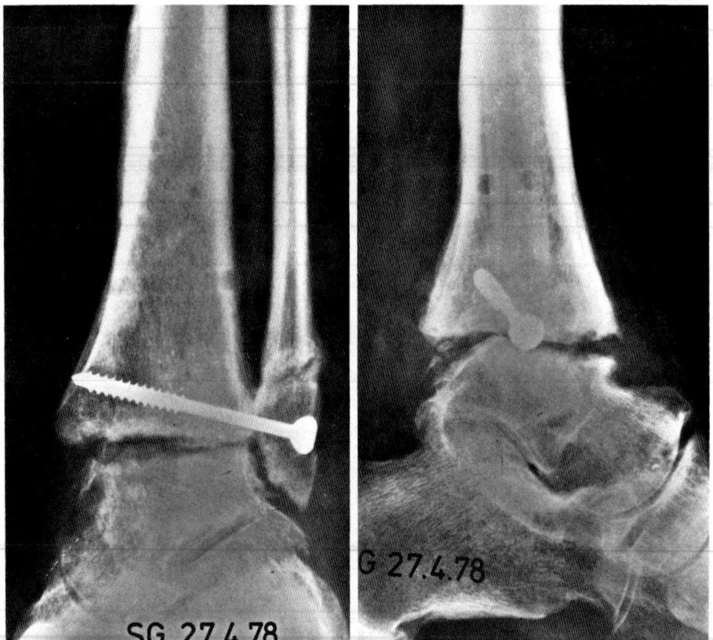

Fig. 86a–d. Stress-locking of Steinmann pins to prevent slippage.
F.H., ♂, age 50, No. 113600.
a Pseudarthrosis after attempted arthrodesis of the ankle joint.
b *Reoperation:* The ends of the two proximal Steinmann pins are moved closer together to stress-lock all three pins and prevent slippage.
c *Five weeks after operation:* On removal of the compression rods, the pins are sufficiently elastic to regain their straight shape. They are now free to be withdrawn.
d *Four months after reoperation:* Arthrodesis consolidated in optimum position

Example 1: Compression arthrodesis of the ankle joint (Fig. 86)

The problem: The Steinmann pins must be prevented from slipping laterally in the bone.

The solution: Adjacent Steinmann pins inserted in a main fragment are stress-locked by moving their ends closer together (compression) or farther apart (distraction). This effectively prevents lateral slipping.

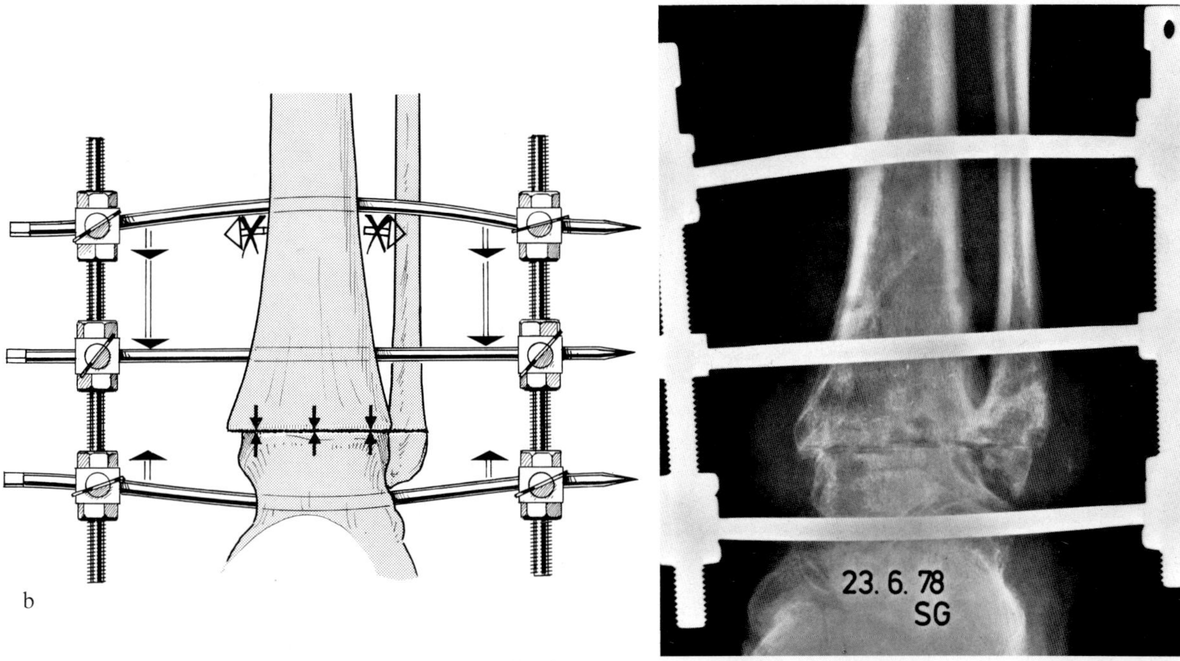

b

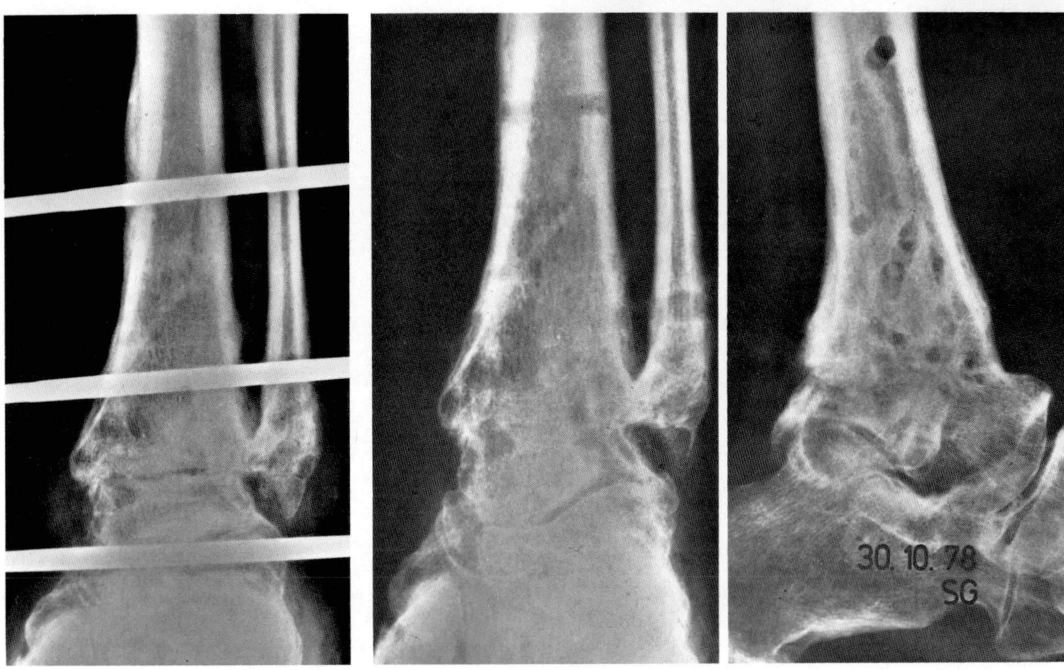

c, d

Example 2: Massive Steinmann-pin traction on the femur (Fig. 87)

The problem: With a traction weight of 20 kg, there is a danger that a Steinmann pin will slip and pull out of the bone.

The solution: The adjacent Steinmann pins are stress-locked in compression with the external fixator. The traction stirrup is attached to both pins, which cannot slip owing to their stress-locked condition.

Fig. 87 a–c. Stress-locked Steinmann pins for traction.
B.S., ♀, age 23, No. 232163.
a Deformity of left hip after infection and removal of a total prosthesis; shortening of limb.
b *Supracondylar traction with 20-kg weight:* The two Steinmann pins are stress-locked and so cannot slip or be dislodged.
c *Ten days after start of traction:* Limb has been lengthened 6–7 cm and is ready for reimplantation of total prosthesis

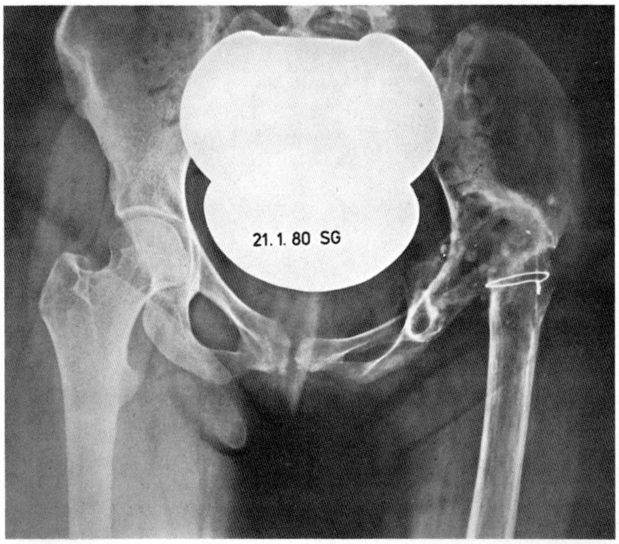

a

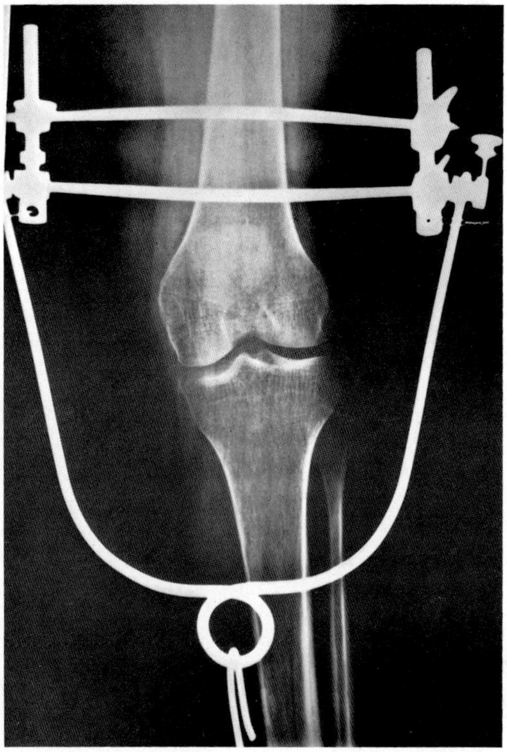

b

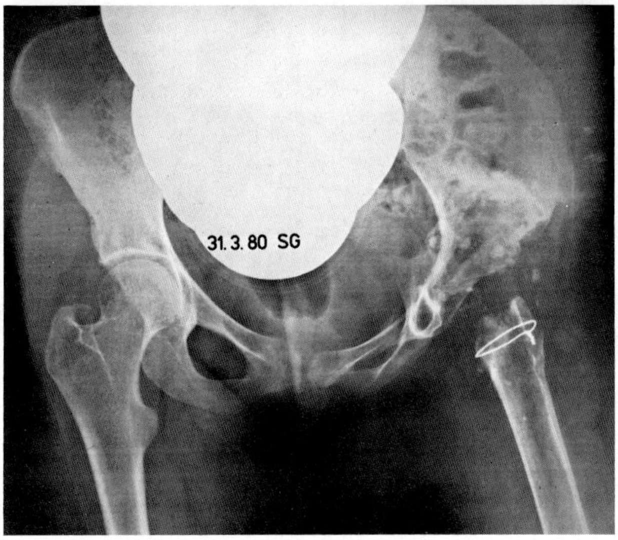

c

Example 3: Valgus tendency in tibial pseudarthrosis (Fig. 88)

The problem: The oblique tibial pseudarthrosis stabilized with the external fixator has a tendency toward valgus angulation.

The solution: A Schanz screw inserted from the medial side exerts pressure on a main fragment, thereby offsetting the valgus tendency while increasing the stabilizing compression in the pseudarthrosis.

Fig. 88a–d. Exerting transverse compression with the external fixator and a Schanz screw.
S.W.A., ♀, age 42, No. 191781.
a Infected tibial pseudarthrosis, valgus deformity.
b *Operation:* Debridement, sequesterectomy, compressive external fixation, decortication, cancellous grafting. The Schanz screw exerts transverse pressure and corrects the valgus angulation.
c *Four months after operation:* Infection healed, pseudarthrosis almost completely healed.
d *One and a half years after operation:* Pseudarthrosis healed in satisfactory position

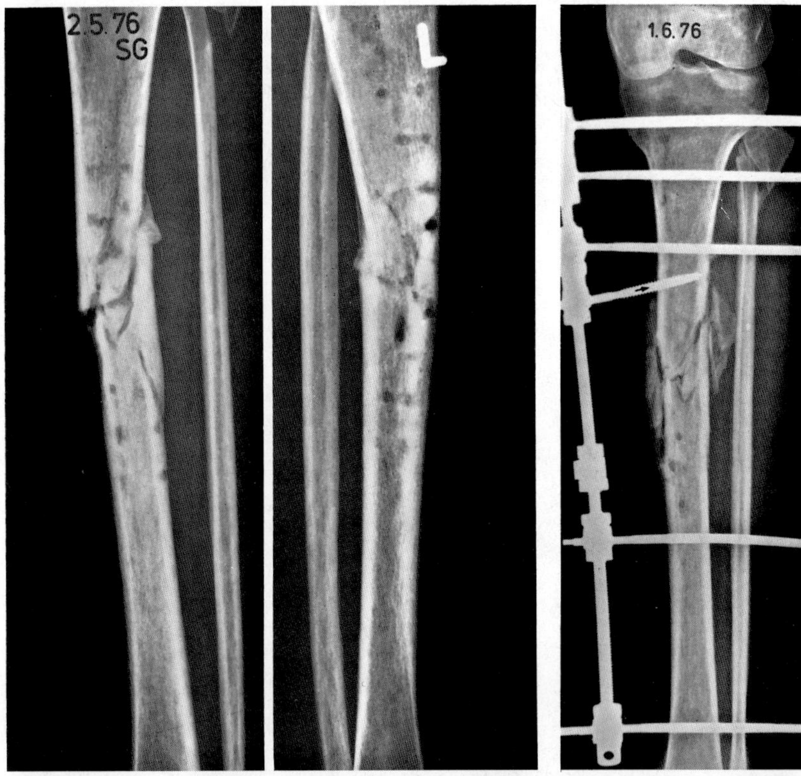

a, b

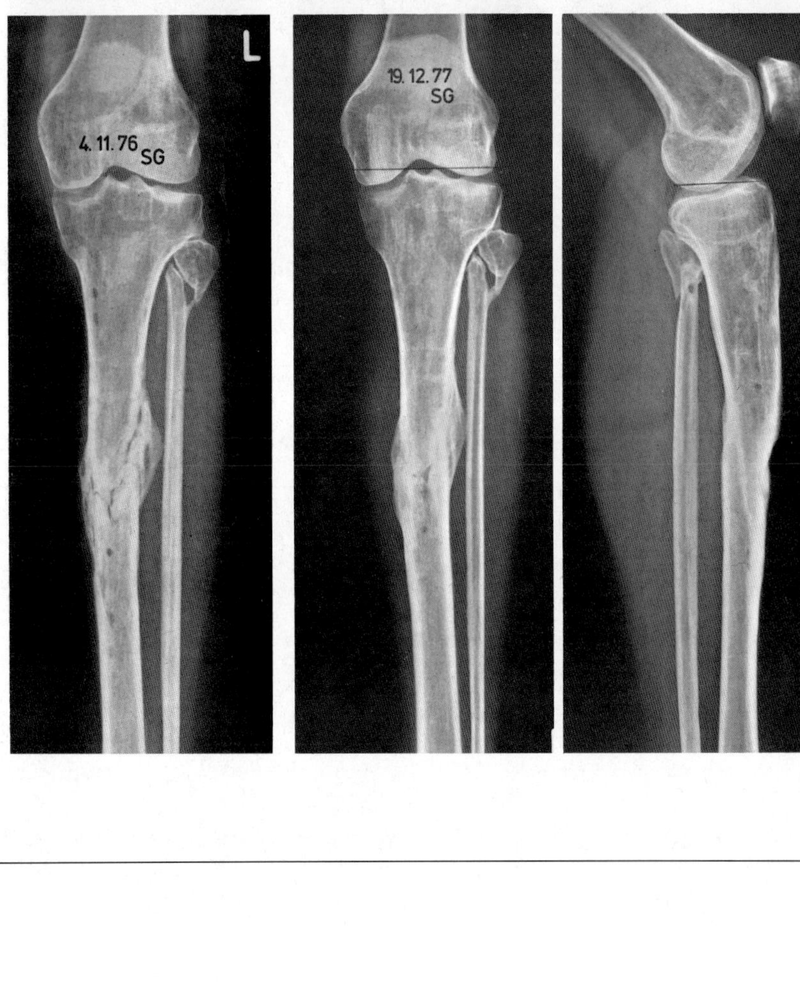

c, d

10.3 Staged Corrections Using the External Fixator

Besides the immobilization of fractures and osteotomies, the external fixator can also be used to effect staged corrections of angular deformities and soft-tissue contractures.

Example 1: Corrective osteotomy of the distal tibia (Fig. 89)

The problem: Every open wedge osteotomy in the distal tibia that is performed in a single stage carries a risk of neurovascular injury caused by the abrupt lengthening.

The solution: To correct the varus deformity, a clamp-type fixator is applied to the tibia. It is used to produce staged distraction until the desired degree of correction is obtained. Then, after an autologous bone graft has been interposed in a second operation, the fixator is switched to compression.

Fig. 89a–g. Staged correction of angular deformity using the external fixator. S.H., ♂, age 16, No. 140420.
a Condition after injury to the epiphyseal plate with faulty and deficient growth. Comparison films: Varus and shortening.
b *Operation:* Application of clamp-type external fixator, slight primary correction.
c *Idea of operation:* During the distraction phase, the bend angle of the Schanz screw is decreased in stages with the aid of bending irons.
d *Two weeks after operation:* Complete correction after daily minimal correction with the external fixator. Now a wedge-shaped bone graft from the ilium is interposed and held fast by switching the external fixator from distraction to compression.
e, f *Six weeks after graft insertion:* Removal of fixator and application of a below-knee walking cast.
g *Nine months after operation:* Corrective osteotomy healed in desired position. Foot has normal trophism and motor function without stretch injury to the nerves, vessels, muscles, or skin

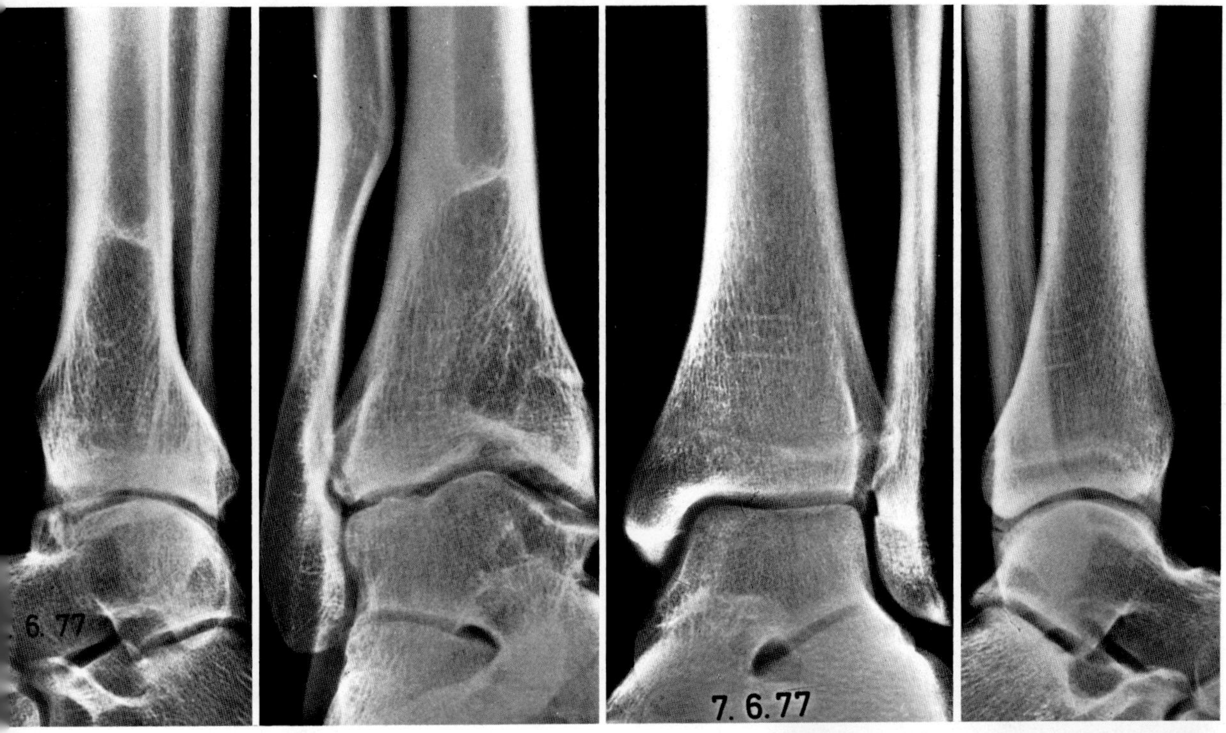

b

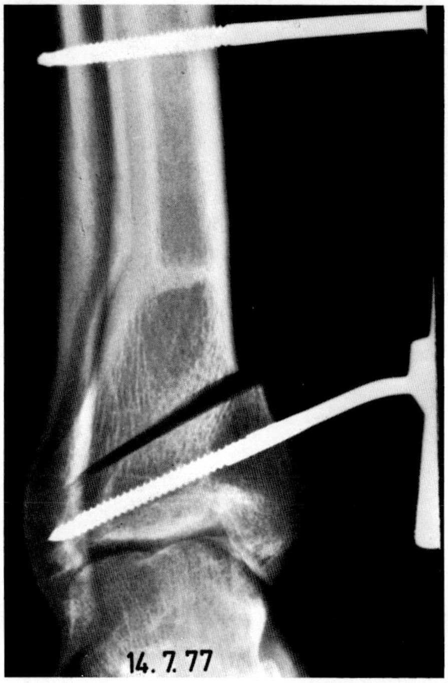

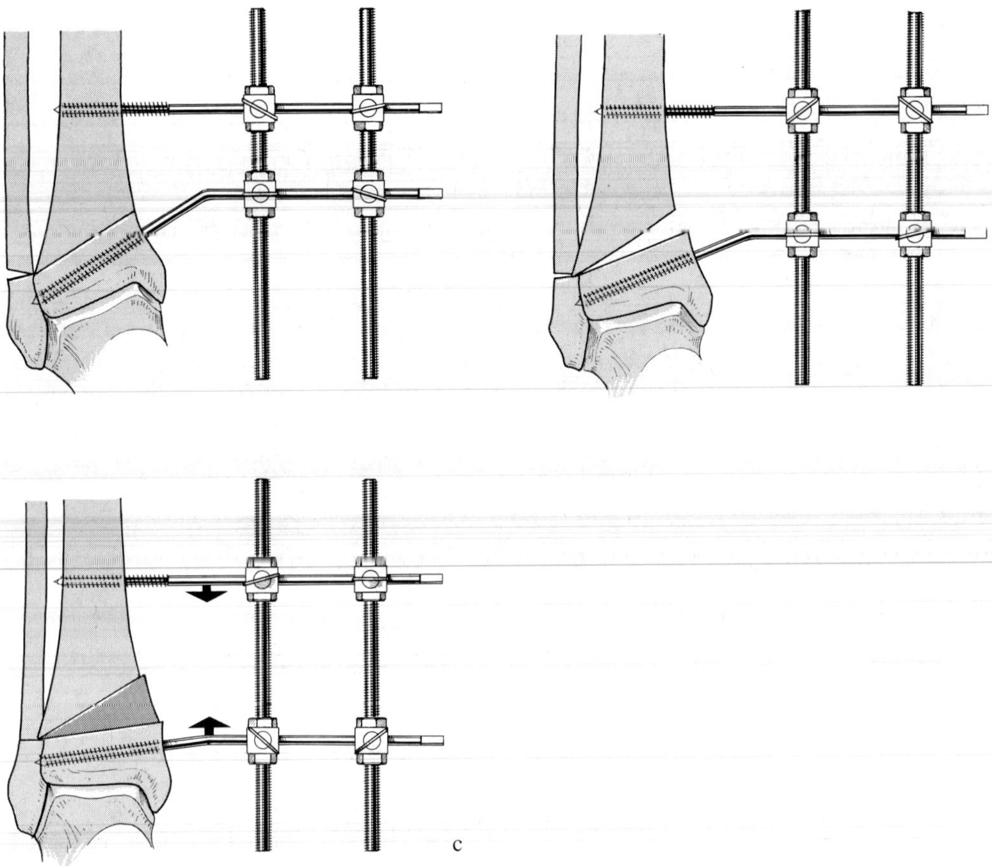

c

Fig. 89c–g. Legend see p. 186

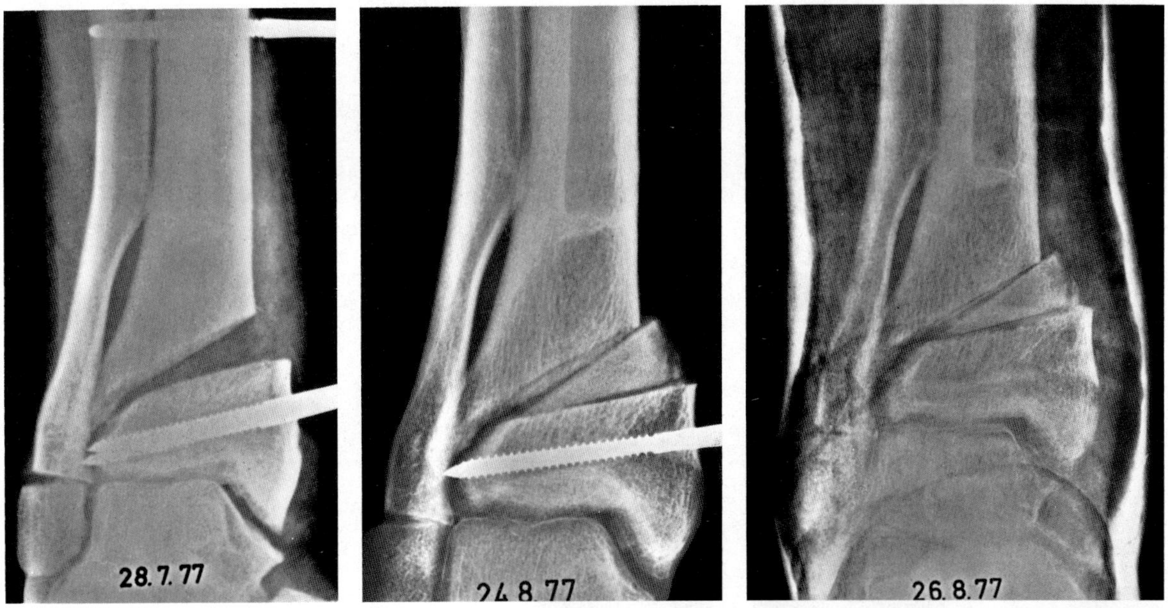

d–f

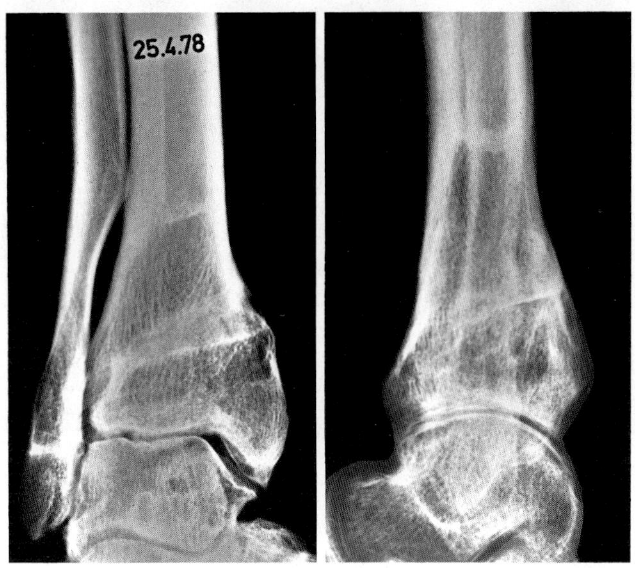

g

Example 2: Post-traumatic equinus deformity with contractures (Fig. 90)

The problem: Post-traumatic equinus deformity associated with peroneus paralysis, posterior tibial syndrome, or prolonged unconsciousness following an injury cannot usually be corrected by Achilles tendon lengthening alone. Unfortunately, section of the tendon does not always give a satisfactory correction, because of associated contractures of a number of other soft-tissue structures.

The solution: One 4.5-mm Steinmann pin is driven through the distal tibia and one through the base of the metatarsals. The pins are interconnected by two external fixation rods. The rods are tightened a few turns each day, effecting a staged correction of the deformity without the need for surgical lengthening of the soft tissues. A separate operative correction may be necessary for clawing of the toes in some cases.

Fig. 90 a–c. Staged correction of equinus deformity using the external fixator.
M.C., ♀, age 14, No. 162042.
a Severe post-traumatic equinus deformity.
b *Schema:* Insertion of Steinmann pins through the tibia and the base of the metatarsals. The arrangement is tightened daily with the threaded rods.
c *Five weeks after start of treatment:* Equinus deformity is corrected

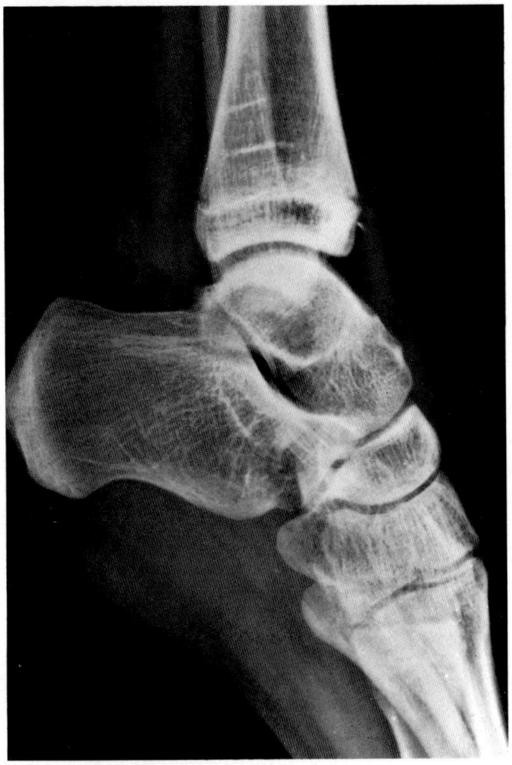

a

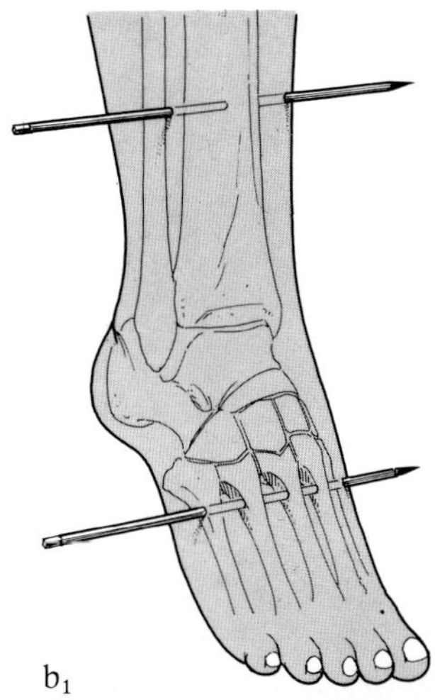

b_1

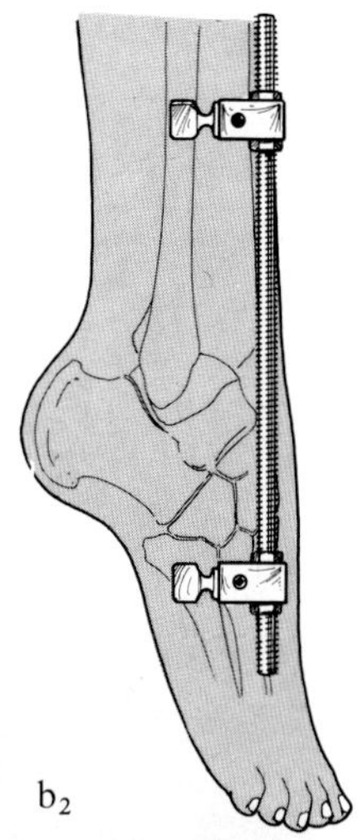

b_2

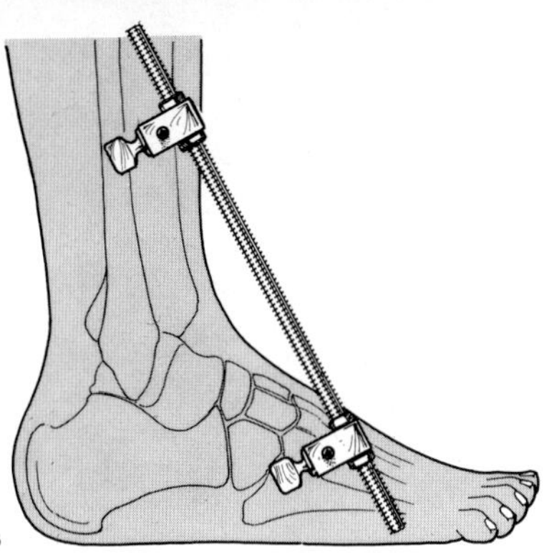

b_3

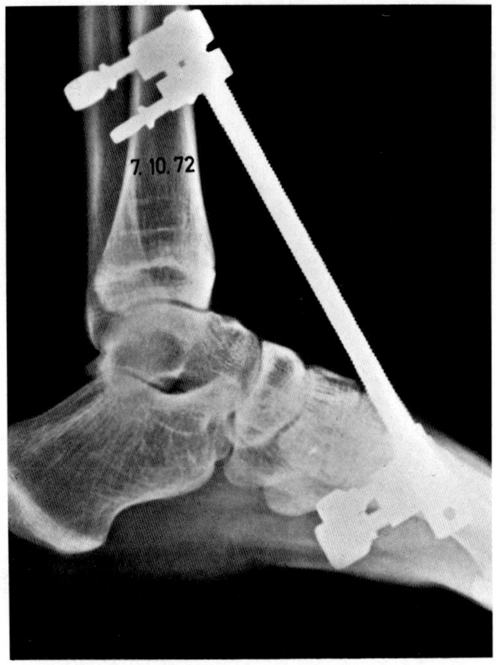

c

10.4 External Fixator for Distraction in a Distal Radius Fracture

In the distal intra-articular comminuted fracture of the radius, there is still some uncertainty as to the proper method of management in the relatively young patient. On the one hand, open reduction of the fracture is difficult because of limited vision of the articular surface. On the other hand, a stable reduction of the fracture cannot be maintained by nonoperative means. The external fixator offers an acceptable solution.

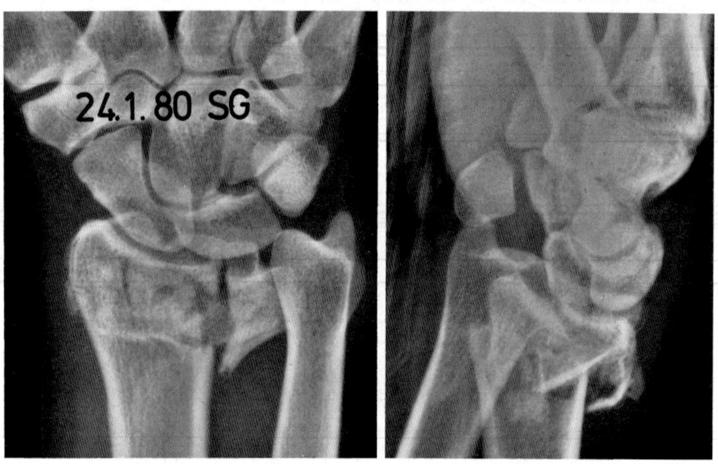

a

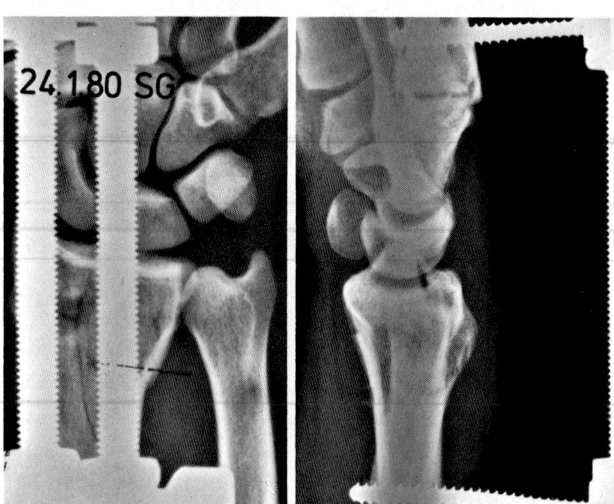

b

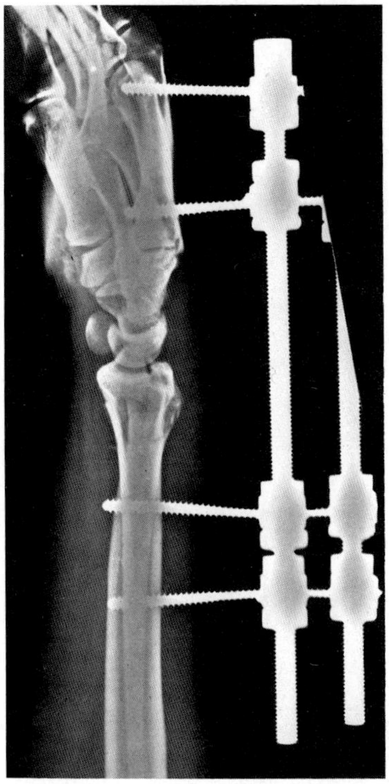

c

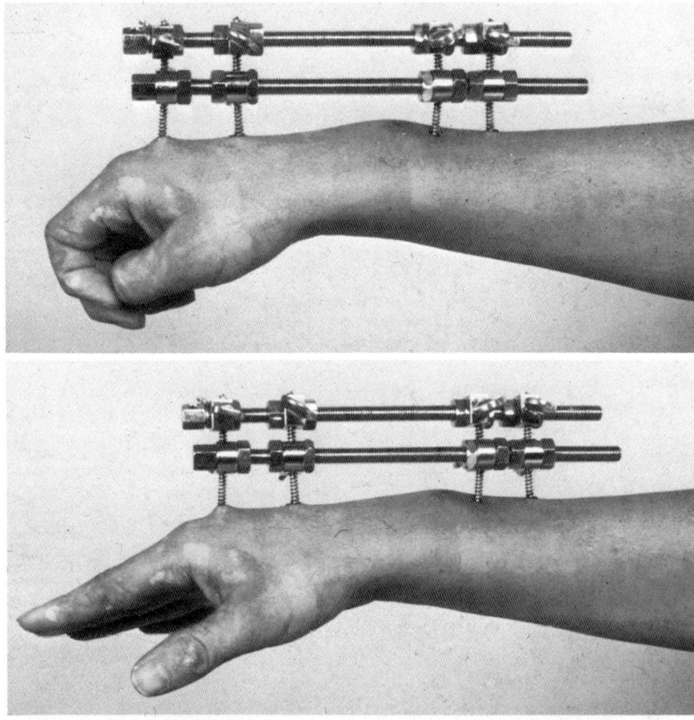

d

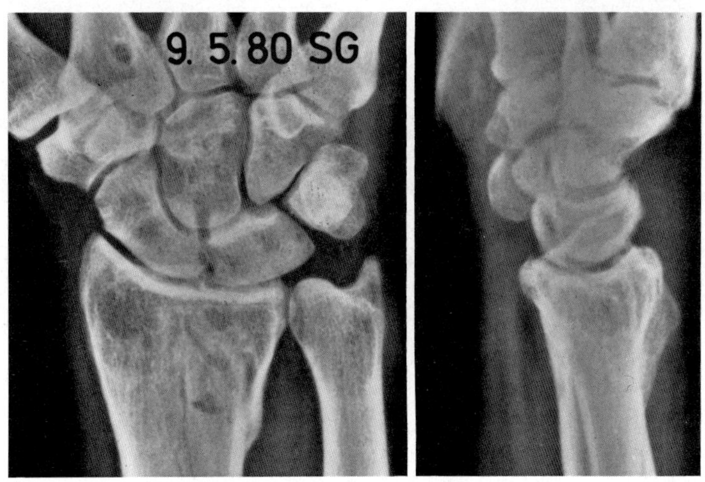

e

Fig. 91 a–e. External fixator for distraction in an unstable fracture of the distal radius.
R. A., ♂, age 29, No. 235882.
a Intra-articular comminuted fracture in a young adult patient.
b Result of closed reduction after application of external fixator.
c *Operative technique:* Two long 4.5-mm cortex screws each are driven into the radius and first metacarpal in such a way that all four screws are in line. One or two threaded rods are mounted onto the screws to serve as spacers.
d No cast is applied, and active exercise is started postoperatively.
e *Three and a half months after injury:* Fracture healed without dystrophy; articular function normal

Example 1: Intra-articular comminuted fracture of the radius (Fig. 91)

The problem: Extensive surgery is necessary for open reduction of the fragments, with a high risk of joint derangement. Conservative treatment is inadequate for a stable reduction.

The solution: An adequate position can be achieved by reduction in distraction and maintained with the external fixator until stable bony union has occurred.

11 Concluding Remarks

The internal fixation techniques described in the *Manual of Internal Fixation* are entirely satisfactory in the great majority of cases. In *Special Techniques* we have attempted to show how unusual problems can often be solved by remarkably simple and straightforward means. We expressly caution the reader that the special techniques presented here are not intended for use in everyday surgical situations.

The importance of giving proper attention to the soft tissues in bone operations cannot be overstated. By the same token, stable skeletal conditions are very often crucial to the healing of damaged soft tissues. Thus it can be seen that internal fixation is an important tool not just for the bone injury itself, but also from the standpoint of soft tissue management. The success or failure of internal fixations reflects an understanding or misunderstanding of this concept, as well as pure technical proficiency, or lack of it, on the part of the surgeon.

It is hoped that this book will further the understanding of the biomechanics of operative fracture care.

12 References

Anderson R (1934) Fractures of the radius and ulna. A new anatomical method of treatment. J Bone Jt Surg 16:379

Anderson R (1945) Concentric arthrodesis of the ankle joint. J Bone Jt Surg 27:37

Blount WP, Clarke GR (1949) Control of bone growth by epiphyseal stapling; a preliminary report. J Bone Jt Surg 31-A:464

Boitzy A (1971) La fracture du col du fémur chez l'enfant et l'adolescent. Masson, Paris

Charnley J (1953) Compression arthrodesis. Livingstone, Edinburgh-London

Danis R (1932) Technique de l'ostéosynthése. Masson, Paris

Danis R (1947) Théorie et pratique de l'ostéosynthèse. Masson, Paris

Hoffmann R (1951) L'ostéotaxis. Gead, Paris

Judet R (1965) La décortication. In: Judet R: Actualités de chirurgie orthopédique IV. Masson, Paris

Lambotte A (1913) Chirurgie opératoire des fractures. Masson, Paris

Magerl F (1979) Die Behandlung von Wirbelsäulenverletzungen. In: Verh Oe Ges Chir Bd II. Egermann, Wien S 859

Magerl F (1980) Verletzungen der Brust- und Lendenwirbelsäule. Operative Behandlung. Langenbecks Arch Chir 352:427 (Kongreßbericht)

Magerl F (1980) Operative Frühbehandlung bei traumatischer Querschnittslähmung. Orthopäde 9:34

Magerl F (im Druck) Clinical application on the thoracolumbar junction and the lumbar spine. In: External skeletal fixation. Williams and Wilkins, Baltimore

McElvenny RT (1957) The treatment of nonunions of femoral neck fractures. Surg Clin N Amer 37:251

McElvenny RT (1957) The immediate treatment of intracapsular hip fracture. Chir Orthop 10:289

Müller ME, Allgöwer M, Willenegger H (1963) Technik der operativen Frakturenbehandlung. Springer, Berlin Göttingen Heidelberg

Müller ME, Allgöwer M, Willenegger H (1979) Manual of internal fixation. 2nd edn. Springer, Berlin Heidelberg New York

Pauwels F (1935) Der Schenkelhalsbruch. Ein mechanisches Problem. Beilageheft Z orthop Chir 63

Phemister DB (1933) Operative arrestment of longitudinal growth of bones in the treatment of deformities. J Bone Jt Surg 15:1

Roy-Camille R, Saillant G (1970) L'ostéosynthèse des fractures du rachis. Fractures du rachis cervical. In: Judet R: Ostéosynthèse. Actualités de chirurgie orthopédique de l'Hôpital Raymond-Poincaré. Masson, Paris

Roy-Camille R, Zerah JC (1970) Ostéosynthèse des fractures du rachis dorsal et lombaire. In: Judet R: Ostéosynthèse. Actualités de chirurgie orthopédique de l'Hôpital Raymond-Poincaré. Masson, Paris

Wagner H (1972) Technik und Indikation der operativen Verkürzung und Verlängerung von Ober- und Unterschenkel. Orthopäde 1:59

Weber BG (1964) Grundlagen und Möglichkeiten der Zuggurtungsosteosynthese. Chirurg 35:81

Weber BG (1966) Operative Frühbehandlung bei traumatischer Paraplegie. In: Rehabilitation der

Para- und Tetraplegiker. Fortbildungskurs Schweiz. Rehabilitationskommission, Bern

Weber BG (1972) Anterior fusion in lumbar disease. In: Orthopaedic Surgery and Traumatology. Proceedings SICOT 620. Excerpta Medica, Amsterdam

Weber BG (1972) Die Verletzungen des oberen Sprunggelenkes. 2. Auflage. Huber, Bern Stuttgart Wien

Weber BG (1974) Knöchel, Fußwurzel, Mittelfuß. In: Chirurgie der Gegenwart, Band IV. Urban und Schwarzenberg, München Berlin Wien

Weber BG (1975) Verletzungen des Hüftgelenkes. In: Chirurgie der Gegenwart, Band IV, Urban und Schwarzenberg, München Berlin Wien

Weber BG (1975) Zuggurtungsosteosynthese mit Draht. Chirurg 46:102

Weber BG (1979) Die Verletzungen des proximalen Femurendes. In: Breitner, Operationslehre IV/2, Ergänzung 33. Urban und Schwarzenberg, München Wien Baltimore

Weber BG, Brunner Ch, Freuler F (1979) Die Frakturenbehandlung bei Kindern und Jugendlichen. Springer, Berlin Heidelberg New York

Weber BG, Brunner Ch, Freuler F (1980) Treatment of fractures in children and adolescents. Springer, Berlin Heidelberg New York

Weber BG, Cech O (1973) Pseudarthrosen. Huber, Bern Stuttgart Wien

Weber BG, Cech O (1976) Pseudarthrosis. Huber, Bern Stuttgart Wien

Weber BG, Magerl F (1975) Fusion of the cervical spine. In: The Arthrodesis, 178. Thieme, Stuttgart

Weissmann SL, Salama R (1969) Trochanteric fractures of the femur. Clin Orth 67:143

Subject Index

E. Letournel, R. Judet

Fractures of the Acetabulum

Edited and translated from the French by R. A. Elson

1981. 289 figures in 980 separate illustrations.
XXI, 428 pages
ISBN 3-540-09875-5

Contents: Surgical Anatomy. - Mechanics of Acetabular Fractures. - Radiology of the Acetabulum. - Diagnosis and Classification. - Posterior Wall Fractures. - Fractures of the Posterior Column. - Anterior Wall Fractures. - Fractures of the Anterior Column. - Pure Transverse Fractures. - T-shaped Fractures. - Associated Posterior Column and Posterior Wall Fracures. - Associated Anterior and Posterior Hemitransverse Fractures. - Associated Both-Column Fractures. - Transitional and Extra-articular Forms. - Associated Injuries. - Distribution of the Clinical Series. - Clinical Presentation. - General Principles of Surgical Management. - Early Treatment of Displaced Fractures. - Treatment of Specific Types of Fracture. - Early Complications of Operative Treatment. - Late Complications of Operative Treatment. - Anatomical Results of Operation Within Three Weeks of Injury. - Clinical Results of Operation Within Three Weeks of Injury. - Surgical Management More Than Three Weeks After Injury. - Reassessment of Patients Treated Before 1971. - Exercises in Radiographic Diagnosis. - Bibliography. - Subject Index.

"The perfect restoration of the articular surface and associated osseous architecture" was the goal set forth by E. Letournel and R. Judet in their surgical treatment of fractures to the acetabulum. Their analysis of more than 300 such cases in "Fractures du Cotyle" showed the usefulness of an appropriate classification system, the importance of careful preoperative assessment of three-dimensional radiographic data, and the need for experience and suitable facilities for successful surgical management of these fractures.
This edition was prepared in response to requests for a similar source of authoritative information for English-speaking orthopaedic surgeons. While the goals and conclusions of the original remain the same, the opportunity was taken to rearrange and expand the text, appending it with selected radiographs for practice analysis. The translation is also enriched with over 250 new cases, as well as follow-up studies of patients reported on the original french edition.

A. Sarmiento, L. L. Latta

Closed Functional Treatment of Fractures

1981. 545 figures, 85 tables. XII, 608 pages
ISBN 3-540-10384-8
Distribution rights for Japan:
Igaku Shoin Ltd, Tokyo

Contents: The Rationale of Closed Functional Treatment of Fractures. - The Scientific Basis of Closed Functional Management of Fractures. - Fractures of the Tibia. - Tibial Condylar Fractures. - Fractures of the Femur. - Fractures of the Distal Radius. - Fractures of the Forearm. - Fractures of the Humeral Shaft. - Delayed Unions and Nonunions of the Tibia. - Fractures in Children.

Functional bracing of fractures is predicated on the belief that function encourages osteogenesis and that absolute immobilization of bone and joints is physiologically unsound and detrimental to fracture healing. The authors have applied the system of functional fracture bracing which they have worked on since 1963 to over 2000 acute fractures of the tibia, femur, radius, ulna, and humerus with a low incidence of nonunion.
In this book, the authors present their system of functional bracing and the extensive research they have conducted in connection with it. Indications and contraindications are given and the step-by-step application of the braces carefully illustrated. The clinical management of various fractures is discussed in the light of representative clinical cases showing the behaviour of various fractures under functional treatment. In addition to diaphyseal fractures, the authors also describe their experiences with Colles fractures, tibial condylar fractures, fractures in children, and delayed and nonunions of the tibia. This unique work will prove a singularly valuable addition to every orthopedic surgeon's store of knowledge. It also includes information of interest to bioengineers, orthotists, orthopedic assistants, and physical therapists.

Springer-Verlag Berlin Heidelberg New York